TRUE FACTS *for the* HEALTHY FAMILY

PATSY WYLIE

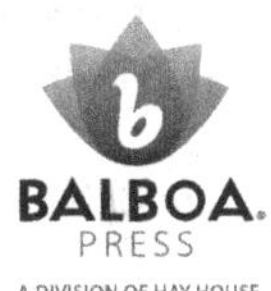

BALBOA PRESS
A DIVISION OF HAY HOUSE

Balboa Press books may be ordered through booksellers or by contacting:

Balboa Press
A Division of Hay House
1663 Liberty Drive
Bloomington, IN 47403
www.balboapress.com
1 (877) 407-4847

Print information available on the last page.

ISBN: 978-1-5043-8832-0 (sc)
ISBN: 978-1-5043-8834-4 (hc)
ISBN: 978-1-5043-8833-7 (e)

Library of Congress Control Number: 2017915092

Balboa Press rev. date: 10/16/2017

This book is dedicated to the many thousand men, women and children who trusted me with their health and wellbeing during weight loss. I want to thank you all very much for the education and life skills you gave to me, I am a better person for meeting and getting to know all of you.

So I thank you very much for that.

Also for my husband Ken who is always with me supporting me in everything I do and my three wonderful children who told me to write this book. Thank you.

Chapter one

Information to help you in selecting the weight loss program that is perfect for you, guiding you through step by step from losing the excess weight and reaching your desired goal weight.

Stabilizing you at your goal and helping you to be able to maintain healthy weight for the rest of your life.

Read all the guidance material; take your time going through it read carefully.

Everything you need is in the book good luck.

Chapter two

Men and weight loss

Chapter three

Getting started

Chapter four

Teaching you how to select the perfect weight loss program

Chapter five

Guidance material that will walk you through your program, helping you to choose the right foods for you during your weight loss

Chapter six

Recipes designed to help you to enjoy what you are doing while losing weight each recipe lets you know what you are getting so as you can put that with the program selections you will have. If you are not a good cook or just have never tried all recipes give you full instructions on how to make it. Good luck

Chapter seven

Guidance material for stabilization and maintaining your goal weight

Chapter eight

Children and weight loss

Very important for those with overweight children; giving you the information you may need to help your child over this hurdle in his or her life. Good luck.

Chapter nine

Obesity a universal problem that needs to be addressed seriously

Chapter ten

Menopause

Chapter eleven

Diabetes: controlling your sugars and managing your weight type 1, type 2 and gestational diabetes & pregnancy

Chapter twelve

Vegetarianism: healthy eating for all types of vegetarianism

Chapter thirteen

Eating disorders giving you the information to help you to understand this very serious and deadly disease that is affecting millions worldwide

I have written this book so as hopefully everyone will understand and be helped whether you are reading for yourself or you are working with others who are going through this. Good luck.

Chapter fourteen

Hypo thyroid and hyper thyroid disease, helping you to understand the difference in these two very different diseases, which afflict millions. Good luck.

Chapter fifteen

GMO's, pesticides, steroids and antibiotics in foods Things you need to know about what you and your family are digesting and what they can cause and are causing all over the world. Good luck.

Chapter sixteen

Mental illness and addiction: understanding drug abuse and addiction

Chapter seventeen

Aspartame: the most controversial food additive in history

Chapter eighteen

Zika virus things you need to know about this very dangerous virus that affects the very young baby in the womb.

Chapter nineteen

Pandas: information about a scary and controversial disorder, behavior brought on by something as common as strep throat in children.

Writing this book I have tried to give you as much information on a multitude of different ailments that most could be avoided, to me prevention is worth a pound of cure. Meaning that if you can prevent something happening you should.

A little about me

I decided to write this book now, and thought what a wonderful way to finish this step in my life.

I have a lifetime of experience, 30 plus years so now I'm going to pass it onto you. Everything you will need to know about controlling your weight, eating properly, helping your children to grow up without health problems and what is in the food that we are eating.

Everything you need will be in this little book.

I was that working mom; I know about being tired, housework, homework, sports, cooking, parties and being the family taxi.

I know very well; bringing home dinner because you're tired, and cooking on top of everything else; well you know. I just thought I'd point that out.

You know writing a book is pretty scary; yet exciting.

I want to write so as everyone will understand. I hope you enjoy and learn everything you need to know.

We are going to go in steps starting at the beginning. When we were children; right up to now as adults. You may relate to parts of this book, and some you will not; but it is for everyone; so I'm covering it all, everything I know you will know.

I wish you all success

Ok let's get started. I have been in the nutritional field for a long time. I'm a certified nutritionist; I have worked with thousands of men women and children. I loved my job, loved the people I worked with, loved to see the happiness just getting healthy did for them. I have worked with both sides of the scale, those who were eating themselves to death and with those who were starving themselves to death. There really is no other way to say it but straight up. So keep reading you probably will find yourself in here. You see our bodies are really the only thing we control. We can be nice to ourselves or nasty.

Over the years I've found that everyone has a problem with their body. We are never happy with ourselves. We either overeat or under eat to solve our problems.

You see we control our bodies it really is the only thing we have full control over. We are always looking for that quick fix. Trust me there isn't one.

You see advertisements all the time on television and internet.

FREE REGISTRATION but really it's not nothing is for free

Why! You have to buy their product in order to start there program so in selling you a product that makes them sales people.

Some of the people they employ to advertise for them are on our televisions; singer's, actors and talk show hosts and we like them! And a few of them have tried just about everything out there with no success; 99% of what they are selling has appetite suppressants in them, these food make you think you are full, wonderful you may say, however, when you stop taking them your appetite comes back with a vengeance. And the cycle begins.

Every time you do something like that you change your body, you speed up metabolism and then you slow it down; not healthy and not good unless you intend to live like that for the rest of your life and believe me that kind of eating gets so boring after a while. They always get so excited about the first 10 lbs. the first 10 lbs is usually fluids in the body; depending on how over weight you happen to be. I'm just being honest with you. I am sure millions of you have tried one thing or another. Just remember be it premade food, protein drinks, or pills they are all the same. People spend billions on weight loss programs every year; and some succeed; but the majority of us don't. There is an old saying (a fool and his money are easily parted) sad but very true.

I know simply because I am a nutritionist, and all of these programs or so called programs have come across my desk.

We are all very good at starting things like painting, knitting and of course starting diets but sticking to it is a very different thing. We make New Year resolutions and say to ourselves this year is going to be different.

Well Rome wasn't built in a day. If you start something with big ideas and then find out it wasn't as easy as you thought it was going to be; if you are not committed to making the change then you won't; you will put it of just like any project that you pick up, saying things like this is not a good week or I'll get back to that next week ETC; don't be too hard on yourself there are millions of us who say exactly the same thing.

Whether you are overweight or underweight both have something in common. We are trying to control our bodies, when we lose control is when we turn to other things, such as alcohol or medication, to make us feel better. This may work for a while but eventually we have to face it.

During my time working in the health field, I have seen and heard many very sad stories; a lot of times I took it upon myself to help people in very sad situations. Saying to myself; there but for the grace of God that could be me.

The worst thing you can do when you start to lose weight on the program is to tell everyone; keep it to yourself: that way you will feel comfortable in all eating situations, and be able to look before you leap.

I have always told my clients that it is no one's business what you do. What I want for you to feel no matter where you are; a restaurant or at someone's home; I want you to feel comfortable and relaxed! Not stressed out about other people; let them notice you; and they will as you lose the excess pounds. Remember when you start to be noticed to say thanks, just eating better, and get on with it. Keep it to yourself until you feel comfortable and confident then you can tell them if you want.

As you read this book everything will become very clear to you chapter after chapter you will be able to follow along. You will learn everything you need to know for yourself and your family. From losing your weight, stabilizing at your goal, and why that is so important; and being able to maintain for the rest of your life. You will teach your family good nutrition and how to eat healthy. You are giving a gift that is priceless. GOOD HEALTH

Weight has a lot to do with self –esteem if we look in the mirror and automatically like what we see then I guess we are ok, however, statistics show more than 85% of the population world-wide thinks very negatively of themselves: That's saying a lot don't you think.

Our bodies are really the only thing we have complete control over, we can either be good to it; or abuse it.

Diet or dieting they are just words; big selling words if you are selling products that say they will make you thin, but what they are not saying is they could also make you sick. If you have children it is very important as to how you behave because they repeat what you are doing and then it becomes a vicious cycle.

A little about doctors and medications; quite a few years back they started to give out pain killers, antidepressants, and yes diet pills like they were in a candy store saying they were not addictive, now they have to eat their words so to speak because they are. When they were testing these medications they the so called researchers said maybe 1% of the population that used a particular drug would get addicted to it. It turns out that was false as 99% that used it did. I personally have seen people who cannot come of the medication because of what it has caused; for example electric shock in the brain, shaking, tremors and loss of memory really horrible for the person that it is happening to.

Quite a lot of doctors have lost their licence to practice over this some have gone to jail. When you go to the doctor and are asked what's wrong with you, meaning you are supposed to diagnose yourself; personally I think there is something wrong with that.

They have got a little bit stricter with the prescriptions, but what they have caused over the years, will in turn take years to correct. How many people do you personally know that are or were addicted to prescription medication, I have met thousands including family members. Ridiculous isn't it.

You may say what has this to do with losing weight absolutely everything; because ignorance is bliss, meaning if you don't know, you can't change it.

You may have to reread this in order to take in what you are reading,

I know I would. I really hope you are learning so you may be able to help others.

Women way back in the day were prescribed valium when they were starting into menopause. "Doctors would say it's all in your head" meaning they were depressed or something. Do you know how many suicides resulted in that or how many became alcoholics and overdosed; millions sickening isn't it.

So as we go along I will be giving you a lot of information some you may need; as you go through life.

Men and weight loss yes we are going to help the males as they too can be sucked into spending a fortune on weight loss products or worse body building products and you know what I am talking about when I say this, so yes I'm here for you too. When men decide to lose weight, it usually has something to do with their health, for example back, shoulder and knee problems, heart problems, high cholesterol and that's just a few. Really I have found that the male usually eats a lot of fast foods, especially if they are left to fend for themselves. Now in saying this it really depends on what they were taught growing up. However, in saying that some men are just lazy; easy is always better and no mess to clean up right!

Stay away from body building supplements and protein powders! If you take a look at the ingredients in supplements and protein powders at most health food stores, you'll find that they contain an array of questionable ingredients, such as aspartame, saccharin, fructose and artificial colors. Interesting to note how unhealthy many of these products really are. Rather than being made with natural ingredients, and sweetened naturally; they are sweetened with chemicals and made with ingredients that are certainly less than healthful. Why you may ask? Because bodybuilders continue to purchase these supplements; in other words, the supplement manufacturers are simply meeting the demands of bodybuilding consumers.

Why are so many body builders so unconcerned with their health? It is something that has been frequently observed in the bodybuilding community: people consuming any products, no matter how dangerous to their health, in order to build more lean body mass and look better for competitions and photo opportunities. This is the case, with the use of illegal steroids for enhancing muscle mass; it is a dangerous trend, not only in terms of steroids but also with protein supplements that contain toxic ingredients such as aspartame.

Let's take a closer look at the problem with aspartame, and see how it affects the human body. In my opinion aspartame should have been banned a long time ago due to its toxicity and potential for nerve damage. When you consume aspartame, it breaks down into two chemical compounds in the human body: formic acid and formaldehyde. Formic acid is an irritant; and does not belong in the bloodstream. The bigger problem here is formaldehyde which is a preservative. This doesn't mean that by consuming aspartame you are going to stop aging. Rather, it means that you are going to suffer the side effects from ingesting this preservative chemical.

Formaldehyde is listed as an environmental toxin by the EPA, and when ingested in the human body it causes widespread nerve damage: damage to the optic nerve, brain cells and the nerve cells. That is why aspartame has been so strongly linked to migraine headaches, muscle tremors, vision problems and mental confusion. These are characteristics that most bodybuilders should hope to avoid. How can you appear healthy if your nervous system is being destroyed by a toxic ingredient you are consuming; I urge bodybuilders and fitness enthusiasts to start reading the labels of the foods, drinks and energy bars they purchase, and check for chemicals sweeteners such as aspartame, sucralose, and saccharin chemical sweeteners should be avoided at all costs.

When men start: like us all we are ready to make the change, easier said than done; but if you make small changes one at a time you will see that you can do anything. Men give up the few things like beer, pop, coolers and the junk food quite easily. They get off track to but once they start to see the difference just a few things make; they usually stick with it and they lose rapidly.

Men and boys need to be motivated, give yourself a pat on the back, and tell yourself how good you will feel when you get the excess weight off. As you are going through your program which is all led out for you in this book. I will walk you through it. I'm with you every step of the way.

Reasons to lose weight = family, health and looks.

When you gain weight you look older, you dress in darker clothes basically to hide yourself, you cut your hair short because you think it makes you look thinner. You get depressed usually start taking anti-depressants which some doctors hand out like candy sound familiar.

You never lose weight for someone else; do it for yourself because you will never make that someone happy when you are miserable. Remember you are the one who is going to look and feel better. If it makes the other person happy because you are that's great; but not important, you are the one that counts.

Being overweight is hard on our health. I don't mean that you get the flu or cold, I mean diabetes, heart disease, problems with our backs, shoulders, knees, hips, high cholesterol, poor sleeping, etc.

We try to fix it with the latest fads be it diet pills, powders, potions trust me they do <u>not</u> work. It can actually make it worse; as you lose weight today and gain it back tomorrow, you are changing the natural rhythm and slowing down your own metabolism. Really what you are doing is hurting yourself. So this is not a diet book. This is a look at yourself book. Let's get healthy together, if you have a family you will all benefit. Have I got your attention yet!

Weight gain is a slow process. We really don't waken up one morning and say oh look at me or do we. It takes time to get fat! May as well say it.

Nothing fits so we put it to the back of the closet saying I'll get back into that;

Really by the time that happens the style may be back, we don't weigh ourselves or look at pictures we move on why because life is busy. I realise that. You have to say enough is enough, for yourself as well as your family.

Remember when you do start to change you are doing it for you first, because if you are doing it for someone else it will not work. Remember it is not selfish to take care of you.

Get ready for a new you. The important thing to keep in mind today is that you will lose weight and become a slimmer, healthier, happier person. You have made a tremendous start. Now, keep going till you reach your goal.

The next few weeks will be filled with excitement and challenges.

Some challenges will come from your old habits and attitudes.

You may experience second thoughts or doubts.

These are normal responses to changing your life'

Resolve now to keep these doubts from interfering with your plans.

Focus on being slender you will succeed.

Other challenges will come from people around you. Some of them think they can second guess you and interfere with your success.

Remember you are in charge of your life. Stay focused on your goal and you will have the last laugh, in just a few weeks you can show them the NEW SLENDER YOU.

You will feel the excitement as you watch the pounds melt away. Shopping will be more fun as you begin to fit into smaller sizes. You will enjoy looking at yourself in the mirror and watching your body take shape.

Friends, relatives, even people you hardly know will tell you how terrific you look. You will have more energy and feel healthier.

You will gain the respect and admiration of others.

Your whole outlook will change and life will seem brighter, because of the commitment you make to-day.

To succeed in your challenge, it is invaluable to have a clear view of your objectives. We are only able to reach that which we clearly seek and that which has not registered as a target may not be attained.

Even if you have had several failures in the past; do not hesitate to establish a new clear and precise goal. Your previous defeats can serve as a means for improvement. Study the reasons that have caused these defeats and take measures not to repeat them.

1. MY OBJECTIVES – write out in order of importance the goals you will pursue, for example; your ideal weight, clothes size it is important to write out what you are aiming for.
2. MY BENEFITS- write out in detail the benefits that will have a bearing on reaching your ideal weight, and how you will profit. For example; to be comfortable with yourself, to be more appealing; to gain self-confidence; to gain personal satisfaction. Note them in order of importance to you.
3. MY SELF IMAGE SEQUENCE- this step is crucial. Our subconscious registers images or impressions, not letters or words. It is said that a picture is worth a thousand words.

Now you must imagine yourself at your desired weight, in clothing and situations that you ardently desire. All the details must be there, your shape, extraordinary sensation of pride and well-being.

This mental exercise must be done every day upon rising and before going to bed. This exercise may take a few seconds to a few minutes. In your diary write out the image you have chosen.

You may stick an old photo of yourself. Be certain to be realistic in the choice of the photo you select. Re-live this image in your mind each day.

"You have to eat properly" in order to be healthy! If you have good health you have everything. So let's get started. First you have to recognise what you are eating, start writing down how you eat, when you eat, and what you are eating daily; and I mean everything. For one week; don't change anything.

Now look over your weekly sheet and see how much starch, fruit, vegetables and protein. What did you drink? Tea, coffee, pop, water, how much alcohol you had in a week, you will be surprised, not with alcohol but with everything.

This week you were learning about yourself. What you choose is what your family eats.

Ok first week is over now let's try my way.

First I want you to step on the scale that you have at home if you don't have one get one as you will be using it, record your starting weight, and say that's the last time I see that number.

Follow the program exactly the way it is written for you it is important for your weight loss as well as your health. Research has shown it takes 21 days for the body to adapt to almost anything; we are not going to shock the system we are going to waken it up gradually. The first seven days I'm taking a few things away, giving you different things to choose from; introducing water into your diet and daily life. This will be you're first week.

The next seven days you will be doing exactly what I have written for you. This is stage two of the program you will either love it or hate it but trust me you will love what you see on the scale; and it only last seven days.

The next seven you are in your weight loss program which you will follow until you have lost the weight and reached your goal. If you follow the way it is designed you will reach that goal. Remember do not play with your program.

MAKE A WEEKLY FOOD DIARY
Day one
BREAKFAST LUNCH DINNER

Start keeping track of your food intake daily this is something to keep you on track of food intake and portion size throughout your weight loss

Stage 1 will be your foundation for a successful weight loss. It is during this phase were you will begin to reduce the elements that have contributed to your weight gain. Follow all of the following directives.

1. Eliminate= in between meal "snacks" (fast foods, pastry, junk foods etc.)
   Instead make some jelly, cut up some fresh fruit and put in large bowl; the only thing that won't keep is banana; so if you like it cut a little up, at any time have 1 cup of jelly and 1 cup fruit. Cut up your favorite vegetables the ones you would choose at a salad bar keep them in the fridge.1 cup un-popped popcorn will fill a bucket take some with you when you are travelling as it will take you where you are going but the nice thing is it will also bring you home meaning you will not be stopping for a snack or drink. To me variety is the spice of life. If you give yourself a good variety you are satisfying a multitude of cravings instead of one.
2. Cut your sugar intake in half, if you take 2 teaspoons you now take 1. Change your salt to sea salt.
3. Salad dressings are another thing. I have found that those who use "fat free" and low fat dressings tend to use more. I prefer to make my own with oil and vinegar then season to your own taste. To make it easier you can use any of the balsamic vinaigrettes some are quite good.
4. All food and beverage consumption should be charted on your food diary.

5. Gradually increase your water intake to eight (8oz) glasses per day. That's a total of 64oz per day.
6. Water is not the no all be all to weight loss if you are eating properly it will assist you in your weight loss, however if you eat poorly it would not matter if you drank two gallons you would expel half and the other you would retain. 64oz is what we need daily whether we are losing weight or not, to keep our body functioning properly.

What is the release point?

As you increase your fluid intake, you will reach a point known as the "release point" at the release point you will notice three signs. (1) A sudden release of the retained fluid. (2) A significant drop in weight. (3) A return to normal thirst.

Most people mistake their thirst for hunger; so instead of giving the body something very natural they feed it instead. My advice to you when you recognise the release point in your body have a glass of water before you eat anything; if you are still hungry after the water then by all means eat!

What is the best way to reach the release point?

Note the amount of water you are currently drinking and continue this for one day. Increase your intake by one 8-ounce glass per day. Keep track of how much water you are drinking each day until you reach the release point.

Remember you will notice a sudden loss of fluid and pounds, and a return of natural thirst. If you then continue to maintain this final level of fluid intake you will enjoy a much smoother weight loss. Pay attention to your thirst!

There will be many days when you will be unable to drink water in accordance with your thirst. It is important to know the number of glasses of water you need to drink so that you can control your fluid level in the event that you have to ignore your thirst.

THE LESS WATER YOU DRINK, THE MORE YOU RETAIN.
THE MORE YOU DRINK THE LESS YOU RETAIN.

Many people think that if they drink less water they will retain less. The body works in exactly the opposite way. When you increase your water intake, your salt supply becomes more diluted and your body stops secreting A.D.H. once A.D.H. secretion is interrupted, your kidneys will adjust by releasing, another reason to keep the kidneys operating at maximum efficiency is that if your kidneys are not releasing fluid and flushing your system of its toxic substances, your body will call upon your liver to detoxify these wastes, to do this your liver will have to ignore some of its other duties.

WATER PILLS

Millions of people are on some form of a water or fluid pill for fluid gathering around the heart, I am not telling you to stop taking it I'm just letting you know the facts of water pills. When you take a water pill you force your kidneys to excrete more salt and water. However, more water than salt leaves your body, and therefore the salt concentration is increased. On the following day your body will retain more water to re-dilute the salt and you will have to continue to take water pills to keep the water off. All you really accomplish with water pills is the loss of many important minerals that are "unnaturally" flushed from your system each day.

SOME OTHER REASONS FOR FLUID RETENTION:

1. Low blood protein as a result of poor protein intake. Often the case for overweight people who move from one fad diet to another.
2. Right before a woman's period there is an imbalance of hormones which results in natural fluid retention.
3. For each pound of carbohydrate ingested, your body will retain three pounds of water.
4. Certain drugs, such as birth control pills, reserpine, cortisone ETC, will cause fluid retention.
5. Sunburn, tension and loss of sleep will contribute to fluid retention.

6. When your body burns 100 grams of fat it produces 120 grams of water. If your cells do not release this water right away, your weight will remain the same. It may even go up. This metabolic level of water release is possible only if your water is proper.

Water is introduced into the body 48% from fluid in the diet, 42% from solids and 10% from the burning of fat tissue.

Water is expelled from the body. 20% from the lungs, 20% from the skin 55% from the kidneys= (urine) and 5% from the intestine= (feces). Whenever solids are decreased in the diet there must be an increase in fluids.

Why do we retain water? The primary cause of water retention is the intake of salt. Salt must be diluted in the body, and so, if your kidneys are holding onto more salt, they need more water to properly dilute the salt. When you eat an unusually high amount of salt, your pituitary releases anti – diuretic, hormones (ADH) signalling your kidneys to reabsorb more water, your urine input goes down and you retain water. These hormones are secreted as needed, and as long as they have sufficient water to work with, your water balance will be maintained.

Why is water so necessary? Did you know that 70% of your body weight is water, and 30% of the total water in your body is in your bones? It is clear that water is a very large and important part of our physical make up. In fact a 20% decrease in the body's water level will result in death! As little as a 10% decrease is considered critical. Water plays an important part in almost every reaction in the body, it is used to transport vital substances to the cells, and it also carries waste products from the cells to the kidneys. Water keeps the membranes of the nose, mouth and respiratory tract well lubricated and facilitates the exchange of oxygen and carbon dioxide in the lungs. Quantities off water are secreted into the intestinal tract to aid in digestion. If the body's water is in short supply, digestion will not proceed normally resulting in constipation. Just a few facts on water I hope this helps you to understand the importance of drinking just 64oz daily.

Medications can enhance or upset your weight loss the pill you may be taking will not make you gain weight, however, how it makes you feel might. Foods that did not tempt you before become more attractive and tempting and you may not notice right away but the medication will not make you gain weight remember that unless of course it is a steroid so be careful what you put in your mouth. The food diary will help you to recognise what you are eating.

The recording of your daily food intake is extremely important to your weight loss for some of the following reasons:

It will make you more aware of what you are eating.

Become more aware of the quality and quantity of the food you are consuming. Self-discipline: Will help you to modify your eating habits and behaviour and improve nutritional knowledge.

Water

1. Rids body of metabolized fat
2. Enhances weight reduction
3. Minimizes problem of water retention
4. Major component of blood and other body components
5. Natural appetite suppressant if used correctly
6. During stage one of program weigh your-self every other day. Monday Wednesday and Friday; while you are losing weight; it is not a good thing to weigh every day as your body needs time to adjust to weight loss.

Take one multivitamin/mineral tablet daily while you are losing weight.

Get water up to 64oz daily.

Two cups regular coffee and tea allowed daily. Anymore should be decaffeinated. Remember cut sugar intake in half.

Ok first week is over, weigh yourself and mark down weight on sheet if you lost 3 to 4 pounds good for you.The next week you will be following what I have written up for you do not replace any food with something else do not stop and start in this stage it is only for seven days you can do it. Millions already have, remember you are not alone.

The first two days are the worst as you may find yourself reaching for something that is not on the list and you will be pulling back. By the third day you will feel more relaxed and prepared for yourself.

Stage two if you have type 1diabetes and using insulin DO NOT follow step 2 of the program as it can cause an unbalance in blood sugars go directly to stage 3 which is your program. Type 2 diabetes you can follow. Children under 13 should not follow stage 2.

STAGE TWO this program cannot be compared to an ordinary diet. By a natural change in your body, this program eliminates your appetite, gives you a sensation of well-being, and makes you lose fat and inches effectively. Your results will be spectacular, but note: one small deviation may cause headaches, dizzy spells, fatigue, 2-3 pound weight gain due to fluid retention and cravings for the next few days. Are you ready?

Eat regularly, at least three meals a day. Eat quantities given not eating enough is just as bad as overeating.

Make sure to avoid salt, sugars, excess carbohydrates and milk products with the exception to those on program. You can use sea salt, balsamic dressing's, and herbs and vinegar spice it up make your food tasty and interesting use your imagination be creative do not be boring with yourself.

Drink 64oz water= eight 8oz glasses every day.

Low impact exercise (walking etc.) 20 -30 minutes, exercise to your own individual tolerance.

When cooking, use oil lightly meaning spray it on instead of pouring.

Remember the consequences of a slight deviation.

Coffee or tea regular 2 cups daily\coffee or tea decaf unlimited

No fruit juices / no cream /no mouthwash/no gel toothpaste just for this week you get it all back when this stage is over so just seven days.

Drink 8oz milk daily you can use this for coffee or tea.

Unlimited daily servings eat until you are full and then push plate away from you as the days go by on this stage you will find yourself filling up much quicker go with that. It is natural you are just finding your full spot.

ENTREES OR PROTEIN = Beef, Veal, Chicken breast, Turkey breast, Fish, Liver and Lamb. (NO SALMON ON THIS STAGE). Special instructions: Entrees must be baked, broiled, micro waved or barbequed. You may eat unlimited portions and servings but only until you are full.

VEGETABLES = Asparagus, Broccoli, Cabbage, Cauliflower, Celery, Chicory, Cucumber, Green beans, Green onions, Lettuce, Parsley and Spinach.

Special instructions: vegetables can be steamed, barbequed, stir fried or they can be eaten raw, do not boil unless you are making soup. You may eat unlimited portions and servings of all vegetables.

One daily serving (OPTIONAL): 1 egg daily/ men can have 2 daily. You can boil, poach or scramble.

Remember if it is not on the list of food you cannot have it on this stage.

As you are going through the program remember to read through what you have written down; your objectives your benefits and your self-image this is how you felt and what you wanted when you started; it's your motivation. Nothing is easy! But I promise you if you follow you will reach that goal honestly you will! Remember you are not alone millions are doing it with you.

Well I bet you're glad that's over; easy right now we will get into your program. I'm going to show you which one you will follow. So starting with your wrist size

Measure your right wrist at the (ulna) smallest part of the wrist. Write it down this is your body frame size.

Between 5inches and 5 ¾ inches = small frame

Small frame height usually between 4ft 8 inches to 5ft 3inches

Between 5 ½ and 6 inches= medium frame

Medium frame height usually between 5ft 4inches to 5ft 6 inches

Between 6 and 7 inches = large frame

Large frame height usually between 5ft 6 inches to 6ft and up

This helps with choosing your program, it also depends on how much you want to lose remember to be realistic with yourself set small goals reach them and move on. Never be disappointed in yourself, remember one step at a time.

General instructions for your weight loss program

Remember. Your program involves; a significant restrictions of calories. Your program has been designed to provide you a balance of calories in the reducing regime. Do not substitute other food which may have the same amount of calories, it may have an entirely different mixture of protein, fat and carbohydrate, which would cause smaller weight loss.

It is important you follow the program precisely to insure the most effective weight loss for you.

Special instructions

Eat three complete meals a day or small amounts as often as you desire do not exceed the required daily servings.

Meat entrees that are high in fat are allowed three times weekly. Never two days in a row.

All portions are raw weight / if you have a large frame they can be cooked weight.

Meat and poultry should be trimmed of all skin, bone and fat before cooking.

Tuna is allowed three times a week, not on the same day you plan on having a high fat meat for dinner. Tuna should be fresh or water packed. Lobster, swordfish, scallops, crab and salmon are allowed twice a week as they are high in sodium. Cottage cheese and yogurt should be 2%

Eggs are limited to four a week.

All vegetables, shrimp, crab and lobster must be fresh or frozen. Do not overcook vegetables as it depletes the vitamins and minerals. You may mix vegetables for a salad. Fruits must be fresh, frozen or water packed, no fruit juices. Fruit should be eaten between meals. Cut your sugar intake in half.

I don't care if you have a pack of gum daily, just don't swallow it.

One lemon per day is allowed, for seasoning or adding to your water.

Seasonings: sea salt, herb Marie, Mrs. Dash, pepper, garlic, herbs, spices, vinegar, juice of one lemon. As you go through your program you will start to mix your own spices you will find out what you like; remember to be creative spice it up never be boring with yourself, try different things you never know you just might like it! no salt or prepared condiments such as mustard or ketchup; if you like mustard buy the dried and mix a tablespoon with a little water add a little honey and garlic; very good seasoning for fish, chicken, pork or beef. Eight ounces of milk daily: to be used in your coffee, tea or in cereal.

Two tablespoons oil is free per day, to cook with or make salad dressings.

Two cups regular coffee or tea per day. Decaffeinated coffee or tea unlimited quantities. Stay away from pop while losing weight as 99% very high in sugar, have a glass of orange juice or apple juice etc. instead just for a change. Remember never be boring with yourself variety is the spice of life.

64oz water daily. Water is in addition to any other liquids allowed. It is necessary to flush waste products from your system.

Be sure to record your total food intake each day, it is necessary to obtain the best weight loss.

I may repeat myself throughout the reason is I want you to succeed.

If you enjoy an alcohol drink have it occasionally my advice is to stay away from beer and coolers while you are losing weight as they will make you retain. A glass of wine or vodka and pineapple or orange juice or rye and water go ahead just remember moderation.

Stage three of program.

Diet plan #1 = 4ft 10 inches to 5ft 3 inches= small to med frame

Daily menu plan
Entrees /protein = 2 servings daily
Vegetables = 2 servings daily
Fruit = 2 servings daily
Starches = 2 servings daily
Fats = 2 servings daily
Milk = 8oz daily
½ cup un-popped popcorn; to snack on morning, afternoon, or evening, whenever you need it.

64oz water daily

Keep a track of foods eaten on your food diary for yourself: That way you will know what you are eating daily. So as not to over-eat or under-eat;

Weigh and measure foods: you need to develop the eye for serving size. I like to think we are ok at home; you can't bring scales to a restaurant or someone's home, when you go out; so being able to look at your plate without saying anything to see if there is too much of one thing and not enough of the other, lets you know what you are going to leave on your plate or what you can have more off.

Don't worry it will get easier and less confusing; as the weeks pass you will have more confidence in yourself and honestly that is the best feeling in the world.

Sample menu diet plan #1 for women

Breakfast
½ grapefruit
½ cup cereal
Lunch
6oz yogurt
Salad mixed veg
1 cup mixed fruit
Dinner
5oz chicken
1 cup vegetables
Breakfast
1 cup mixed fruit
½ cup cereal
Lunch
5oz cottage cheese
Salad
Orange
Dinner
4oz fish
1 cup vegetables
¼ cup cooked rice
Breakfast
½ banana
½ cup cereal
Lunch
2 eggs
Salad
½ pita
Dinner
3.5oz beef
Orange
1 cup vegetables

8oz milk daily & 64oz water

Stage three of program

Diet plan #2 = 5ft to 5ft 6 inches = small to medium frame

This plan is designed for women who are 250lbs to 350lbs or more; in order to decrease foods and make it easier to lose weight, as you lose excess and get below 200lbs change program to diet plan #1 and continue with it until your goal weight is reached. I have found this is the perfect program to help with this. No shock to the body, and gives you the chance to adapt to weight loss in a healthy way.

Daily menu plan
Entrees or protein = 3 servings daily
Vegetables = 4 servings daily
Fruits = 3 servings daily
Starch = 2 servings daily
Fats = 2 servings daily
Milk 8oz daily

½ cup un-popped popcorn to snack on morning, afternoon, or evening whenever you need it.

Water 64oz daily

Keep a track of foods eaten on your food diary for yourself: that way you will know what you are eating. So you don't over-eat or under-eat. Weigh and measure foods. You need to develop the eye for serving size. I like to think we are ok at home; you can't bring the scales to a restaurant or someone's home, when you go out. Being able to look at your plate without saying anything to see if there is too much of one thing and not enough of another, lets you know what you are going to leave on your plate or what you can have more off.

Don't worry it will get easier and less confusing; as the weeks pass you will have more confidence in yourself; and honestly that's the best feeling in the world.

Stage three of program

Diet plan #3 for women =5ft 4 inches to 6ft tall = medium to large frame

Daily menu plan

Entrees or protein= 2 servings daily
Vegetables = 4 servings daily
Fruit = 3 servings daily
Starch = 2 servings daily
Fats = 2 servings daily
8oz milk daily

½ cup un-popped popcorn to snack on morning, afternoon or evening, whenever you need it.

64oz water daily

Keep track of foods eaten on your food diary for yourself: that way you will know what you are eating daily. So as not to over-eat or under-eat; weigh and measure foods: you need to develop the eye for serving size. I like to think we are ok at home; you can't bring the scales to a restaurant or someone's home, when you go out. So being able to look at your plate without saying anything to see if there is too much of one thing and not enough of another, lets you know what your are going to leave on your plate, or what you can have more off.

Don't worry it will get easier and less confusing as the weeks pass; you will have more confidence in yourself; and honestly that is the best feeling in the world.

This meal plan is ideal, for men 5ft to 5ft -7inches; and medium to large frame, and are= 210lbs to 350lbs; follow this until you are 200lbs and then change to diet plan #4 and follow it until you reach your desired goal weight.

This will help you to adapt comfortably and have a much more consistent weight loss.

Follow food quantities on male program as you will need larger portions.

SAMPLE =FOOD DIARY DIET PLAN # 3 / 8oz milk daily and 64oz water

Breakfast
½ grapefruit
½ cup cereal

Lunch
6oz yogurt
Salad
1 cup mixed fruit

Dinner
5oz chicken
2 cups vegetables
1/ pita
1 orange

Breakfast
1 cup mixed fruit
½ cup cereal

Lunch
5oz cottage cheese
Salad
Orange

Dinner
4oz fish
2 cups vegetables
¼ cup cooked rice
1 cup watermelon

Breakfast
½ banana
½ cup cereal

Lunch
2 eggs
Salad
½ pita
½ cup pineapple

Dinner
3.5oz beef
Orange
2 cups vegetables
Stage three of program

Diet plan #4 for male's = 5ft 7inches to 6ft and taller = large frame

Entrees or protein = 2 servings daily
Vegetables = 4 servings daily
Fruit = 3 servings daily
Starch = 4 servings daily
Fats = 2 servings daily
Milk 8oz daily

½ cup un-popped popcorn to snack on morning, afternoon, or evenings whenever you need it.

64oz water daily

Keep track of foods eaten on your food diary for yourself: that way you will know what you are eating daily so as not to over-eat or under-eat; weigh and measure foods: you need to develop the eye for serving size. I like to think we are ok at home; you can't bring the scales to a restaurant or someone's home when you go out. So being able to look at your plate without saying anything to see if there is too much of one thing and not enough of another, lets you know what you are going to leave on your plate, or what you can have more off.

Don't worry it will get easier and less confusing as the weeks pass; you will have more confidence in yourself; and honestly that is the best feeling in the world.

There are three steps to weight loss in order for you to maintain your goal weight for the rest of your life naturally. Your first step is reaching your realistic goal weight, the second will be stabilizing yourself at your goal, and the third is maintaining your weight. Don't worry I will be with you every step of the way.

Sample=Food diary male program #4 8oz milk daily and 64oz water

Breakfast
1 cup mixed fruit
1 cup special k

Lunch
6oz yogurt
Large salad
Peach

Dinner
6oz chicken breast
2 cups vegetables
½ cup cooked rice
Kiwi

Breakfast
2 poached eggs
2 slices rye bread
1 cup mixed fruit

Lunch
Large salad
1 cup watermelon

Dinner
6oz white fish
2 cups mixed vegetables
Orange
2 small potatoes

Breakfast
1 cup mixed fruit
1 cup special k

Lunch
6oz yogurt
Large salad
Apple

Dinner
5oz beef
2 cups vegetables
1 cup watermelon
2 small potatoes

FOOD GROUP SELECTIONS = FEMALE

Proteins --------- servings daily

Restricted foods

The following meats are high in Fat and limited to three times weekly.

Beef
Chuck roast = 3.5oz
Flank steak = 3.5oz
Ground sirloin = 3.5oz
Round steak = 3.5oz
Rump steak = 3.5oz
Sirloin steak = 3.5oz
T-bone steak = 3.5oz
Veal
Cutlet = 3.5oz
Filet = 3.5oz
Rump = 3.5oz
Pork
Shoulder = 3.5oz
Loin = 3.5oz
Leg = 3.5oz
Loin chop = 3.5oz
Poultry
Chicken (dark, no skin) = 3.5oz
Turkey (dark, no skin) = 3.5oz
Moose
Venison = 3.5oz
Lamb = 3.5oz
Liver
Beef = 3.5oz
Calf = 3.5oz
Chicken = 3.5oz
Fish: The following is restricted to twice weekly.
Tuna (water packed) = is allowed three times weekly =4oz

These are your high-fat choices while losing weight so remember to weigh and measure servings; for portion control when you are eating out.

Dairy and egg protein exchanges
Tofu = 5oz
Cottage cheese 2% = 5oz
Yogurt = 5oz
Eggs (medium) = 2 maximum of four eggs weekly; while you are losing weight
1 egg +2.5oz cottage cheese
Each one of these equals 1 serving of protein instead of meat
Milk = 8oz daily

<u>Unrestricted foods</u>
The following are lower in fat; and can be eaten daily.

Poultry
Chicken breast (no skin) = 5oz
Turkey breast (no skin) = 4oz
Fish
Arctic char = 4oz
Bass = 4oz
Bluefish =4oz
Cod = 4oz
Grouper = 4oz
Haddock = 4oz
Halibut = 4oz
Orange Roughy = 4oz
Perch = 4oz
Red snapper = 4oz
Shrimp = 4oz
Sole = 4oz
Trout = 4oz
Whitefish = 4oz

Fats ___________ servings daily

Margarine, butter, miracle whip, olive oil, corn oil or sunflower oil;

Serving for each = 1 teaspoon.

These are your low fat choices of protein while you are losing weight; remember to weigh and measure.

FOOD GROUP SELECTIONS = VEGETABLES, FRUIT AND STARCHES
FOR MALE AND FEMALE PROGRAMS

Vegetables: -------- servings daily:
Asparagus – raw = 1 cup – steamed = 1 cup
Beans (wax, green, yellow or string) - raw= 1cup- steamed = 1 cup
Broccoli – raw = 1 cup – steamed = 1 cup
Cabbage – raw = 1 cup – steamed = ¾ cup
Cauliflower – raw = 1 cup – steamed = 1 cup
Celery – raw = 1 cup – steamed = 1 cup
Chicory – raw = 1 cup- steamed = 1 cup
Cucumber – raw = 1 cup- steamed = 1cup
Eggplant – raw = 1 cup – steamed = 1 cup
Fiddleheads – raw= 1 cup – steamed = 1 cup
Lettuce – raw = 1 cup – steamed = 1 cup
Mushrooms – raw = 1 cup – steamed = 1 cup
Parsley – raw = 1 cup – steamed = ¾ cup
Peppers – raw = 1 cup – steamed = 1 cup
Radish – raw = 1 cup – steamed = 1 cup
Spinach – raw = 1 cup – steamed = ½ cup
Tomatoes – raw = 1 cup – steamed = ¾ cup
Zucchini – raw = 1 cup – steamed = 1 cup

The next group of vegetables get smaller in portion size; the reason for this is that these can react as a vegetable or starch in the body. The sad thing is you do not know until you eat them. So watch for your body's reaction.

Alfalfa sprouts – raw= ½ cup – steamed = ½ cup
Bean sprouts – raw = ½ cup – steamed = ½ cup
Brussel sprouts – raw = ½ cup – steamed = ½ cup
Carrots – raw = ½ cup – steamed = ½ cup
Green onions – raw = ½ cup – steamed = ½ cup
Green peas – raw = ½ cup – steamed = ½ cup
Leeks – raw = ½ cup – steamed = ½ cup

Mixed vegetables – raw = ½ cup – steamed = ½ cup
Onions – raw = ½ cup – steamed = ½ cup
Parsnips- raw = ½ cup – steamed = ½ cup
Pumpkin – raw = ½ cup – steamed = ½ cup
Squash – raw = ½ cup – steamed = ½ cup
Turnips – raw = ½ cup – steamed = ½ cup
Fruits ------- servings daily

Apple = 1 small
Apricots = ½ cup
Banana = ½ medium
Blueberries = ½ cup
Blackberries = ½ cup
Cantaloupe = ½ cup
Cherries = 10 medium
Currants fresh = ½ cup
Grapes = 12 medium
Grapefruit = ½ medium
Honeydew melon = ½ cup
Kiwi = 1 small
Mandarin orange =1 large
Mulberries = 1 cup
Orange = 1 small
Papaya = ½ cup
Peach = 1 small
Pear = 1 medium
Pineapple = ½ cup
Plums = 2 small
Raspberries = ½ cup
Rhubarb = 1 cup
Strawberries = 12 small
Tangerine = 1 medium
Watermelon = 1 cup

Remember to weigh and measure vegetables and fruit; to train your eyes for portion control.

Starches ------------ servings daily

Farina enriched = ¼ cup
Diet bread = 2 slices
Melba toast (unseasoned) = 2 slices
Melba rounds = 4 rounds
Rice cakes (unsalted) = 1 cake
Cream of wheat (dry weight) = ¼ cup
Porridge (dry weight) = ¼ cup
Dried cereals = ½ cup
Shredded wheat = 1
Bran (100% all) = 1/3 cup
Red river = ¼ cup
Special K = ½ cup
Soda crackers unsalted = 3 squares
Arrowroots = 1 piece
Brown / or rye bread = 1 slice
Popcorn (air-popped) = 1 cup
Rice (cooked) = ¼ cup
Potatoes = 1 medium
Pasta (cooked) = ½ cup
Pita mini = 2 slices
Pita regular = ½ slice
White bread = ½ slice

Potato pasta and rice: there is nothing wrong with them; it's what we add on top that adds fat to the fire. Mix them with the vegetable you are going to have; that will make your plate that much more interesting.

Remember to weigh and measure food!

FOOD GROUP SELECTION =MALE

Proteins---------- servings daily
Restricted foods: The following meats are high in fat and are limited to Three times weekly:

Beef
Chuck roast = 5oz
Flank steak = 5oz
Ground sirloin = 5oz
Round steak = 5oz
Rump steak = 5oz
Sirloin steak = 5oz
T-bone steak = 5oz
Veal
Cutlet = 5oz
Filet = 5oz
Rump = 5oz
Pork
Shoulder = 5oz
Loin = 5oz
Loin chop = 5oz
Poultry
Chicken (dark no skin) = 5oz
Turkey (dark no skin) = 5oz
Moose
Venison = 5oz
Lamb = 5oz
Liver
Beef = 5oz
Calf = 5oz
Chicken = 4oz
Fish = the following are restricted to twice weekly:
Crab, Lobster, Salmon, Scallops and sword fish: = 4oz
Tuna (water packed) three times a week =4oz

These are your high fat choices while losing weight; remember to weigh and measure; to help you develop portion control when you eat out.

Dairy and egg (protein exchange) male
Tofu = 5oz
Cottage cheese 2% = 6oz
Yogurt = 6oz
Eggs =2 medium
1 egg + 2.5oz cottage cheese = equivalent to 1 meat serving
Maximum four eggs weekly
Milk = 8oz daily

Unrestricted food: The following foods are lower in fat and can be eaten daily.

Poultry
Chicken breast (no skin) = 6oz
Turkey breast (no skin) = 6oz

Fish
Arctic char = 6oz
Bass = 6oz
Bluefish = 6oz
Cod = 6oz
Grouper = 6oz
Haddock = 6oz
Halibut = 6oz
Orange Roughy = 6oz
Perch = 6oz
Red snapper = 6oz
Shrimp = 6oz
Sole = 6oz
Trout = 6oz
Whitefish = 6oz

Fats ----------- servings daily
Margarine, butter, miracle whip, olive oil, corn oil or sunflower oil:
Serving for each = 1 teaspoon

These are your low fat protein choices; while you are losing weight: Remember to weigh and measure

TIPS TO HEALTHY EATING

CHECK YOUR GARBAGE

Do you always eat all those nutritious fruits and vegetables you buy: or do you just buy them with good intentions? Make sure to use them as snack foods to curb cravings or eat a salad before your meal – this will help to make you feel fuller.

THREE OR SIX MEALS DAILY YOU DECIDE

You don't have to eat three large meals a day. You will be more satisfied eating six small meals a day because you won't find yourself hungry or craving, therefore you will be less likely to deviate from you program.

EATING OUT- DON'T WORRY

Most restaurants prepare low –calorie foods. Make sure to ask for dressings on the side that way you are in control of how much you use. Make sure meats are baked, broiled or barbequed, with no additives.

Also, you don't need to eat everything on your plate, take some home.

FOR YOUR INFORMATION

The following fruits and vegetables are great thirst quenches and extra refreshing since they are loaded with water: water- melon 93%,

Strawberries 90%, grapefruit 89%, cucumber 95%, lettuce 94-96%, Bell pepper 95% cut some up; have it to snack on.

ADD VARIETY

Our body needs more than forty different nutrients a day, and no one food group supplies them all. Therefore, make sure to add variety to your meals, you'll also find it easier to eat healthy when you don't eat the same foods over and over again.

LABEL MANIA

Are you checking food labels for what it doesn't have – like cholesterol, salt, sugar and fats, also think of buying food for what it does have – like minerals and protein?

DON'T GO HUNGRY

Starvation or skipping meals is no method of weight management. Usually people who do skip meals tend to have more trouble controlling their weight.

Eat regularly and eat enough to feel satisfied but not stuffed.

TEMPTING FOODS SHOULD BE HARD TO GET

Keeping high calorie low-nutritious foods like candy bars, chips and cookies on hand is too tempting. If you give into cravings easily, leave those foods at the store, you'll think twice about having to go out to get them.

BEHAVIOURAL GUIDANCE MATERIAL

Part One

Fat free foods are less satisfying than the real thing, so we tend to eat more of them. Ironically many of these products have just as many calories as their Full-fat counterparts. Follow this rule: if you wouldn't eat the full fat product, don't, indulge in the fat-free version either.

Don't drink all of your fruit opt for fresh fruit rather than juice. A piece of fruit gives you the satisfaction of chewing, takes longer to consume, and helps you feel fuller because it's loaded with fiber. Plus it's lower in calories than fruit juice.

Limit your alcohol consumption. It can reduce your body's ability to burn fat. It also tends to encourage overeating since alcohol can cause you to lose control.

Limit alcohol consumption to two or three drinks per week.

At the table make meals melodic, listen to slow music at mealtime. It can help you take smaller bites, chew longer and eat slower.

Fool your eyes. Serving food on smaller plates will help you feel satisfied with recommended serving size and not over-eat. Count to three. Want to make food truly satisfying! Focus on the first three bites and chew them carefully.

Stop cleaning up. Break the bad habit of eating until your plate is clean by purposely leaving a few bites untouched at every meal. Eventually, it will feel natural to stop eating when you are full and not when your plate is empty.

Enlist the troops. Ask your family to help you put away extra food after meals, so you will not be able to pick at the left overs in private.

PERSONAL CONTROL GUIDE -CHANGING YOU'RE EATING HABITS

Part One

Most overweight people have specific eating habits which could be improved upon. Since these are "habits" it is easy to ignore them and gradually put on some extra pounds. Over weight individuals frequently feel that they are eating like anybody else, and they are amazed when they notice they have gained weight. What usually happens though is that these people are no longer even conscious of how these poor eating habits cause them to over eat. It is very important that you become more aware of how you are eating so you can change these habits. Since this is so critical, this topic will be divided into two weekly guides. Make sure you refer to these suggestions frequently, because it will take a good deal of time and effort on your part to unlearn those old habits and build new ones.

SLOW DOWN YOUR EATING

There are several problems associated with eating quickly. One problem is that, by eating fast, your food does not have time to settle in your stomach and signal that you have eaten enough. You therefore eat more than you normally would if you were eating more slowly and giving your food time to digest. Another disadvantage with eating too quickly is that you don't have a chance to savor your food. You again end up eating larger quantities of food to get the same satisfaction, which could be derived from a much smaller quantity. This can be done in a variety of ways.

CHEW YOUR FOOD WELL

Many people do not even seem to chew their food. It is difficult to understand how somebody can enjoy their food when it is almost swallowed whole. You will find eating a much more pleasurable experience if you chew your food thoroughly and become more aware and sensitive to the taste of it. Also never take another mouthful while you still have food in your mouth. Chew what is in your mouth and swallow it before taking any more. You will eat less and enjoy more.

TAKE SMALLER BITES

Research has shown that overweight individuals tend to take larger mouthfuls of foot than thin people. A person may not even be aware of doing this. By taking larger mouthfuls of food, however, it is easy to consume larger amounts of food that you are aware. You will find that it is much easier to limit yourself if you cut food into smaller pieces and take smaller portion in each mouthful. Again, you will find how satisfying relatively small quantities of food can be.

BEHAVIOURAL GUIDANCE MATERIAL

Part Two

Have all or none. For some people, it's actually easier to pass up a favorite snack food entirely than to limit themselves to just a taste. When faced with can't – eat-just –one goodies, tell yourself that even though you can have them, it's just not worth it.

Work around weak moments, don't just plan your snacks ahead of time prepare them. For instance, put a healthy treat on the counter or in the fridge before you go out the door. It's the best insurance against a bad snacking decision when you get home.

Single size it. Use little plastic bags to separate snack foods into-one –serving size portions. That way you won't be able to devour the entire box at one sitting. Read to lose; When the urge to eat strikes, pick up a good book. Reading is a great non-food related activity. It's also interesting and comforting, which is good for those who eat when they are bored or stressed. Drink before you eat. It's common to mistake thirst for hunger and eat when what your body really craves is fluids. So hydrate first before you reach for food.

Eating out edicts; know before you go. Decide what you are going to eat ahead of time; (at least have a general idea). If you're familiar with the restaurant, don't even look at the menu. Pick a pricey dish. It provides instant portion control. Restaurants can afford to serve oversized amounts of less-costly items, such as pasta and chicken, but they tend to scrimp on more expensive foods; choose shrimp of filet mignon. Place the first order. Listening to everyone else's choices makes it too tempting to change your mind.

Take your time reading your guidance material they really will walk you through all stages of your program. Remember they are facts not fiction.

Part Two

Hopefully you have noticed some changes in some of your eating habits. As you probably noticed, many of these old habits are don't almost automatically and it takes a considerable amount of persistence and determination to learn them.

This week we will be moving on to some other methods of eating more effectively. It is essential, though; that you do not forget about the ones you practiced last week.

MAKE SMALL PORTIONS SEEM LARGE

There is considerable research in the psychological and perceptual factors that influence peoples eating. A large quantity of food which is placed on a very large platter appears smaller than it really is. If you are eating off this platter, you are likely to eat more than you would normally. The reverse of this principle is also true however, and you can make that work for you. To do this, buy some plates which are significantly smaller than your present ones and use them regularly. This has the effect of making even small portions of food appear larger than they are in reality. You thereby minimize the chance that you will overeat; because your eyes were bigger than your mouth, careful and attractive placement of food on your plate can give you the impression that there is more than there actually is.

DO NOT BE A "CLEAN YOU'RE PLATTER"

Many overweight people grew up in families where leaving food on your plate was almost a crime. You have probably heard the "the people starving in china" routine which is designed to make you feel guilty for not eating everything in front of you. The problem with this sort of reasoning, however, is that starving people in china are not being helped by an overweight Canadian who overeats. Despite this poor reasoning, a large percentage of overweight people persist in plate cleaning; even though they have had enough to eat. Even a few extra bites at each meal in order to clean your plate, has been shown to cause several pounds of extra weight each year. Make a point of leaving some food on your plate every time you sit down to a meal. Do this even if you are not filled up at the end of the meal. By doing this, you make it much easier to leave food on your plate when you are filled up. Do not fall prey to the belief that you are wasting food. You are being far more destructive, especially to yourself, by forcing down unnecessary food.

Part Three

Ban the bread basket. If your companions don't mind ask that the bread basket be removed from the table. When you are out to dinner; or else just move it out of your reach. Eat before you go. Have a snack before going to a cocktail or dinner party. This will help you to control your appetite once you are there.

Your best bet is a combination of complex carbohydrate and protein, such as 3oz yogurt and an apple.

Don't make open ended offers. Instead of asking what you can bring to a party, volunteer a specific food you know you'll be able to eat. Fruit salad, low-fat desserts and crudité are always welcome dishes.

Do the opposite. Use your non-dominant hand when handling finger foods at parties. You'll be surprised at how much slower and less you will eat.

Never go empty handed. Keep your hands full, but not with food. With a drink in one hand and your purse in the other, you won't have any fingers free for food.

Make your smile sparkle. Brush your teeth right after a meal, to signal the end of eating and help prevent post meal picking.

Keep your kitchen in the dark. Clean up immediately after a meal and turn of the kitchen lights. A dark spic and span room should cancel thoughts of snacking.

Sleep well. The more regular and restful your sleep the more manageable your hunger and food cravings will be. Too little sleep usually leads to eating more, especially foods high in sugar and fat.

Food fixes. Dress for success store salad dressing in a spray bottle. You'll save tablespoons worth of fat and calories by spritzing instead of pouring it on.

EXTERNAL CUES

Most people, whether overweight or not, are influenced by the sight, smell and taste of food as well as a variety of other food related stimuli. The sight and smell of a fancy piece of pastry in a bakery window; is frequently sufficient to lure even the best intentioned passerby inside. Research shows, however, that people who are overweight tend to be even more influenced by these external cues, than there thin counterparts. In these cases, the overweight individual is no longer eating out of hunger, but rather because of external stimulation.

Eating in this manner is learned, however, there are several specific measures which you can take to make sure that these external factors do not control you're eating.

AVOID OVERLY ATRACTIVE FOODS

Most food companies are very skilled in the preparation and packaging of their foods. Many foods and snacks seem almost irresistible to some people. These ate the foods to avoid! Do not even purchase those especially attractive foods which entice you to eat regardless of your state of hunger. Every person has those items which are "weaknesses". Become aware of those and make sure they do not get into your house; because they are powerful external initiators of eating.

OUT OF SIGHT- OUT OF MOUTH

It is a fact that many people are much more likely to eat those foods which are visible than those which ate not. Therefore, keep a lot of tinfoil on hand as well as other non-transparent food wrapping materials. Instead of keeping foods in clear-wrappers, re-wrap them in something which will not allow you to see what is inside. In doing this, you avoid this sort of "external" eating by eliminating the possibility that you will eat food merely because you see that it is there.

Part Four

SHOW ME THE WAY

Researchers say that it takes an average of 21 days of practice to develop a new habit. In your effort to permanently change you're eating and exercise routines, keep a positive attitude. Instead of focusing on how terribly you used to eat, and how out of shape you are, concentrate on how happy, fit and energetic you will feel once you have shed your old attitudes towards diet and exercise. If you can dream it, you can do it.

FADS + MYTHS = CONFUSION

Even though modern science inevitably unveils the truth behind fads, the myths just the opposite! These cuts are tender; but they have the highest fat content. Funny that they are the most expensive too; meat marked "select or good" are typically lower in fat. How about this one: yogurt is a health food! Isn't necessarily so! Some fruit on the bottom yogurts and frozen yogurts contain more sugar than a chocolate bar, and, whole milk yogurts are high in fats.

Your best plan is plain, non-fat yogurt with fresh fruit. Non- dairy creamers and whipped toppings are low-fat alternatives to cream? Oops! Wrong again! Non -dairy does not mean low-fat. Often these products contain highly saturated fats like palm and coconut oils (and many are loaded with sugar). The best choice for a coffee whitener is evaporated milk.

ALCOHOL

In addition to supplying "empty" calories (no nutritional value whatsoever) another problem that alcohol causes for those trying to lose weight is that, since it is absorbed quickly into the blood, blood sugar rises rapidly. To compensate, the body secretes insulin. Insulin is a fat-hording compound. It actually makes less fat available for the body to burn as fuel. So if you feel like a guilt-ridden slug after gulping down your sixth brew in two hours, you should! Because in the battle to lose fat, you've just helped out the competition- you've assisted on the goal scored by the mighty fats!

SHOW ME THE WAY

"I feel like eating, so I must be hungry". Actually, you might not be. Thirst, stress, boredom, anxiety and fatigue are often mistaken for hunger; and why fill the tank when it's still ¾ full? If you're not truly hungry try drinking a glass of water or a glass of orange juice, going for a walk, or taking a nap before succumbing to the fridges beckoning. If you find that you're obsessed by overpowering cravings, like the ones that some people have for chocolate indulge a little and then get on with healthy low-fat eating. Or better yet, try sensible, appropriate alternatives. For instance, when it comes to satisfying your cravings for chocolate covered almonds; a bag full of celery and carrots. Sticks just won't cut it. However, chocolate pudding made with 1% or a fudgsicle might do the trick.

People are used to eating fat. It has a pleasing sensation in the mouth that is hard to resist, even though most people are coming to realize the health benefit of cutting back. But making healthy food choices does not mean you have to sacrifice the pleasures of eating. There are a million ways to make delicious and extremely flavorful low-fat foods-foods that your taste buds will fancy and foods that you will start to crave instead of fat-laden choices. Mouth feel is something that can change gradually. Just because you want to be a healthy eater doesn't mean you want to enjoy your food any less, right.

When you don't have the time or the ingredients to prepare homemade macaroni and cheese, you can transform the boxed variety into a creamy low-fat version by making a few changes (use the cheese packet and macaroni as directed). Instead of ¼ cup of butter & ¼ of 2% milk, try ¼ cup sour cream & 3 tbsp. of milk. No one will know the difference and you'll save an incredible 375 calories and 45 grams of fat.

One package of macaroni & cheese, prepared as directed on box weighs in at an unthinkable 1230 calories & 60 grams of fat. 49% of its calories are derived from fat!

BEHAVIOURAL GUIDANCE MATERIAL

Part Five

SHOW ME THE WAY

Fat is undoubtedly a dietary scoundrel when over-consumed but believe it or not, fats not so bad once you get to know it. It does have redeeming qualities too. In fact, we need a certain amount of fat to survive. Dietary fat supplies us with linoleic acid, an essential fatty acid which is important growth, especially in children. Fat is also the vehicle that transports fat-soluble vitamins (A, D, E AND K) through the body and is required for the maintenance of healthy skin and for the metabolization of cholesterol. So eating a low –fat diet doesn't mean eating no fat, and it doesn't have to mean never eating a high fat food. Expect that you will have cravings for chocolate or a T-bone steak every now and then, treat yourself, and then get back on track, with low-fat choices for the rest of the week.

QUESTION: What can add inches to your physique even though it's empty?

ANSWER: "empty" calories like the ones in alcohol. Alcoholic beverages provide calories and nothing else (except the occasional great beer commercial). If you drink regularly- two beers or two glasses of wine per day – that's about 1400 calories per week, or more than 73,000 calories per year, enough to create approximately 20 excess pounds of unsightly flab! And it's highly unlikely you'll burn of any of those extra calories.

JUST REMEMBER TO ENJOY YOUR VICES IN MODERATION

Holidays are often the time that willpower is weakest. When you have "visions of sugar cookies dancing in your head", who can think of eating anything low in fat? Most of the time, one little indulgence or mistake leads to the attitude "oh who cares! I've blown it already, so I might as well really pig out"! It is very important to realize that one mistake or one high fat, high calorie occasion doesn't mean you've blown it. It's the next 2,500 fat laden calories do the most damage. It's easy to devour six "oh" what the heck shortbread cookies and a cup of eggnog in less than two minutes, but they'll hang around on your waistline for a lot longer than that! Remember that eating well isn't all or nothing. It's what you do consistently over the long haul that counts.

Part Six

A FEW FACTS ON EXERCISE OR WORKING OUT

The moment I decide to stop lifting weights, my muscle will start turning to fat!

Muscle is muscle, fat is fat. So don't be afraid to add weight training to your exercise regimen as a way to tone and strengthen your body.

What you do to-day is very important. After all, you're exchanging a day of your life for it!

Forget the slogan "no pain no gain"

Pain is often an early warning sign of injuries from strain and overuse. But killer workouts (working out at an intensity that's leaps and bounds above your normal fitness level) can damage more than just muscles, tendons and ligaments. More damage is ultimately done to your attitude about exercise in general, and your desire to make it a regular part of your life. Who looks forward to voluntary torture? Who would want to stick with it? No –one that's who! It makes much more sense to exercise at a moderate, consistent level for a longer period of time than it does to get in there and act like a Ninja Turtle on a sugar high. When planning their daily activities, people often don't make time for exercise because they place it in the play\ recreation category, making it seem unimportant. Now, let's think about this for a moment. Is it important to be healthy and energetic? Is it important to feel good and to look good? Is having self-esteem and self- confidence something that matters to you? Is sleeping well important? The answer to all of the above questions is a resounding YES, and these are just some of the reasons why people should do some sort of healthy physical activity every single day. Putting exercise higher on the priority list is a good first step towards a healthy, energy filled life.

People who are already thin don't need to exercise! No weigh! Everyone needs exercise every weight, every age everyone! Exercise does more than just burn calories; it strengthens the heart and lungs, lowers the risk of disease, increases immune system functioning helps us sleep well and relieves depression and stress. You don't need to exercise if you don't care about being healthy, physically fit or looking and feeling good; and if you don't care about these things, then what exactly do you care about,

ATTITUDE IS A LITTLE THING THAT MAKES A BIG DIFFERENCE.

Part 6 Page 2

Recipe for fitness and good health =

1. Combine large muscle groups into active units.
2. Stir in a variety of enjoyable activities. Mix them up.
3. Blend moderately and continuously for at least 30 minutes(caution: extending time to 45 minutes to 1 hour may result in severe burning of fat
4. Store leftover energy for use the next day, as process should be repeated at least 3 times a week. ENJOY.

Like the booster shots your school nurse gave you as a child, exercise can be considered another form of "immunization" against illness and disease. Studies show that moderate and consistent exercise, such as walking for a minimum of 30 minutes a day at least four or five days a week, protects us against cardiovascular disease, high blood pressure, depression and anxiety. It reduces body fat and the risk of diabetes and colon cancer, boosts the immune system functioning and increases bone mass.

The only exercise some people get is; jumping to conclusions, running down their friends, side stepping responsibility and pushing their luck!

Cellulite: those unsightly dimples. If you're thinking of using creams, pills or injections to "spot reduce" in areas where plenty of cellulite lives, you should hold onto your wallet- its contents are all you would be losing. You can't spot reduce fat, no matter where it is. Getting rid of the cellulite look involves the same process as reducing fat anywhere else on the body: cutting back on the fat you eat: and getting some regular exercise, a healthy varied diet along with exercise minimizes overall body fat, allowing the underlying muscle to show through. Throw in some weight or resistance training and the appearance of your muscles will improve further. You can't eliminate fat from a certain part of your body by exercising that part alone. Your body can't selectively draw from fat stores in parts being exercised; it draws on fat from all areas. So don't waste your time on pills, potions, creams or schemes to fight cellulite. Just move it! Nature gave us two ends- one to sit on and the other to think with. Our success depends on which one we use the most. Round and round you go. It's a vivacious circle. Physical activity sets of a chain of events that keep you coming back for more. The more active you are the more energy you have, the better you feel, the more you want to do. Getting on the right track is as easy as that.

For your information:
Just the facts about fats!

We're faced with different types of fat in our diets, and each has a different effect on the body (mostly ill effects). Research suggests that two types of fat are good for us, although they are beneficial only when eaten in moderation. Our best bet is to find ways to eat less of all types of fat.

<u>SATURATED FATS=</u> is solid at room temperature and then turns to oil when heated. Most saturated fats are animals in origin, derived from meat, poultry and dairy products (butter, cheese, milk, cream and eggs). It is wise to limit intakes of foods that contain saturated fats. They tend to raise cholesterol and triglycerides levels, and studies indicate that they seem to interfere with immune functioning. Coconut oil and palm kernel oil are high in saturated fat even though they are plant oils.

<u>POLYUNSATURATED FATS</u> = originates from plant sources and is liquid at room temperature. They're considered to be a "healthier" fat because they help lower total cholesterol and triglyceride levels. Vegetable oils such as safflower, sunflower, sesame, cottonseed and corn oil are polyunsaturated fats.

<u>MONO UNSATURATED FATS</u> = includes olive oil, canola and peanut oil. Oils that are high in monounsaturated fats are the "healthiest" choice of oil, as they help decrease the levels of L.D.L (the bad cholesterol).

<u>HYDROGENATED FATS</u> = starts out as liquid fats but is solidified when hydrogen atoms are added. In essence, a healthy fat (unsaturated)

is converted into an unhealthy fat (saturated) some nutritional tricks that add to the profit margins of food manufactures. Why the magic show? Hydrogenated oils give products longer shelf lives since the oil is less likely to break down over time and become rancid. Most of the hydrogenated fats we eat come from partially hydrogenated vegetable oils which are commonly found in packaged foods such as cookies, crackers, snack foods, sauces, pastries and muffins as well as margarine, shortening, peanut butter and deep fried foods. Needless to say hydrogenated fat shouldn't be taken "lightly". Read the label before you buy.

TRANS FATS:

Tran's fat: an unhealthy substance, also known as Tran's fatty acid, made through the chemical process of hydrogenation of oils. Hydrogenation solidifies liquid oils and increases the shelf life and the flavor stability of oils and foods that contain them. Tran's fat is found in vegetable shortenings and in some margarine, crackers, cookies, snack foods and a lot of other foods.

Tran's fats are also found in abundance in "French fries". To make vegetable oils suitable for deep frying, the oils are subjected to hydrogenation; which creates Trans fats. Among the hazards of fast food, "fries" are prime in purveying Tran's fats.

Tran's fats wreak havoc with the body's ability to regulate cholesterol in the hierarchy of fats, the polyunsaturated fats which are found in vegetables are the good kind they lower your cholesterol. Saturated fats have been condemned the bad kind. But Tran's fats are far worse. They drive up the LOL (bad) cholesterol, which markedly increases the risk of coronary heart disease and stroke. According to a recent study so some 80,000 women and men for every 5% increase in the amount of saturated fat a woman or man consumes; his or her risk of heart disease increases by 17%; but only a 2% increase in Tran's fats will increase his or her risk of heart disease by 93%!

The FDA way back in 1999 proposed that the nutrition facts labels on vegetable shortenings and some cookies, crackers, margarine and other foods should carry information about trans fatty acids, or trans fats. Beyond information about Trans- fatty acids or Trans- fats in the food: The FDA rule would also define them "Trans- fat free" and limit the use of certain nutrient or health claims related to fat content, such as "lean" and "low saturated fat". Well it's 2016 and we are still waiting. When something stays fresh for longer that it should; that should tell you something.

In the realm of dietary dangers, Tran's fats rank very high. It has been estimated that Tran's fats are responsible for some 50,000 early deaths a year in the USA. World-wide the toll of premature deaths is in the millions.

Bottled bacteria recycle; but don't reuse.

With every purchase of a bottle of water, you can expect to pay around $1.50, an expense that can add up over time, in fact, you are doing your wallet and the environment a favor by reusing your bottle right? Wrong. Recycling your bottled water can pose risks to your health.

Dangerous bacteria and toxic plastic compounds have been found in the types of water bottles that are typically reused in schools and workplaces nationwide.

One of the toxins that frequently appeared in water samples from reused water bottles was DEHA (diethyl hydroxylamine), a carcinogen (cancer causing agent),

Regulated in drinking water; because it has been found to cause weight-loss, liver problems and possible reproductive difficulties. A study conducted by Cathy Ryan of the University of Calgary found bacteria in elementary schools water bottles that would prompt officials to issue boil advisories, if the water came from a tap.

Researchers discovered bacterial contamination an about a third of the samples collected from the reused bottles. Even carefully washing your bottle is not enough to rule out safety concerns. Research conducted by a graduate student at the University of Idaho suggests that the kind of thorough washing that could kill bacteria might make the bottle unsafe in other ways.

Single-use water bottles are commonly made of plastic called polyethylene terephthalate (PET), which is found to break down over time.

The study found that frequent washing might accelerate the breakdown of chemicals from the plastic, potentially causing chemicals from the plastic to leak into the water.

Both the Canadian and international bottled water associations (IBWA) recommend these bottles for a one time use only.

A water filter on your own tap at home would be a lot safer. Or just use your own water at least you know what you are drinking.

Difference between sea salt and table salt

Though mainly sodium chloride, sea salt and table salt are different from each other, both with respect to the way they are obtained from nature and their nutritive value. Sea salt is considered to be more beneficial for health as compared to table salt, due to over 80 nutritive substances present in it. Read on to know the differences between sea salt and table salt.

The importance of sea salt in human life can be gauged by the fact that the romans paid their soldiers sea salt as their wage. It is from this practice that the word "salary" had its origin. Almost 75% of our body is made up of water. However, this water in not in its pure form, it has salt dissolved in it that helps in a number of functions of the body.

Salt present in the cells and tissues of our body helps in muscle contractions, proper conduction of nerve impulses and transport of nutrients into the cells. Salt may be obtained from sea water or may be mined from underground deposits. Table salt, sea salt, kosher salt and iodized salt (which are a form of table salt with iodine added to it) are the four main types of salt available to us.

SEA SALT

Sea salt is the unrefined salt that is obtained by simply evaporating the water from the seas or oceans. Sea water is channelled into man-made pools along protected shores, and is then left under the sun till all the water gets evaporated. What is left behind in the pools is sea salt. Sea salt is 98% sodium chloride, while the remaining 2% is made of other important minerals like iron, magnesium and other trace elements. Due to higher mineral content, sea salts are more flavoured than table salt.

TABLE SALT

The common table salt is 99.9% sodium chloride. It is obtained from the terrestrial salt deposits which are mined, heat blasted and chemically treated. Due to these processes, table salt is stripped of all minerals other than sodium and chloride. Some anti-caking agents are added to table salt to make it free flowing. Although, initially table salt which had just sodium and chlorine as the only minerals was consumed by people, later on, salt manufactures started adding iodine to it to prevent people from suffering iodine deficiency diseases.

TABLE SALT Vs SEA SALT

Besides the difference in the manufacturing process, sea salt and table salt differ in the following ways: while sodium and chlorine are the only minerals contained in table salt, sea salt has other minerals like iron, sulphur and magnesium naturally present in them. This increases the nutritive value of sea salt as compared to table salt. The various minerals present in sea salt helps us to maintain a healthy balance of the various electrolytes in the body.

The refining process of table salt strips it of all of its minerals, other than sodium and chloride; this makes it an unnatural substance as compared to sea salt, and contributes to high blood pressure, heart and kidney disease. On the other hand health benefits of sea salt, include, proper sleep, promoting efficient working of the liver, kidneys and the adrenal glands. Sea salt also boosts the immune system of the body and will not cause high blood pressure like refined table salt.

You decide what you want to put into your body, personally I use sea salt always have and always will.

Water

We all know that water is important what you are reading; as you read this book is fact not fiction so read it carefully for yourself as well as your family.

75% of us are chronically dehydrated (likely applies to half the world population) 37% of us; the thirst mechanism is so weak that it is often mistaken for hunger. Even mild dehydration will slow down one's metabolism as much as 3%. One glass of water shuts down midnight hunger pangs for almost 100% of dieters. Lack of water is the #1 trigger of daytime fatigue. Preliminary research indicates that 8-10 glasses of water a day could significantly ease back and joint pain for up to 50% of sufferers. A mere 2% drop in water can trigger short term memory, trouble with basic math and difficulty focusing on the computer screen or on a printed page. Drinking 5 glasses of water daily decreases the risk of colon cancer by 45% plus it can slash the risk of breast cancer by 79% and one is 50% less likely to develop bladder cancer. Interesting yet not on the news!

Again this is a fact not fiction.

Now we look at coke

No wonder it tastes so good.

1. In many states in the USA the highway patrol carries two gallons of coke in the trunk to remove blood from the highway after a car accident.
2. You can put a T-bone steak in a bowl of coke and it will be gone in two days.
3. To clean a toilet pour a can of coke –cola into the toilet bowl and let the "real thing" sit for one hour, then flush clean. The citric acid in the coke removes stains from vitreous china.
4. To remove rust spots from chrome car bumpers: rub the bumper with a crumpled up piece of Reynolds wrap aluminum foil dipped in coke-cola.
5. To clean corrosion from car battery terminals: pour a can of coke-cola over the terminals to bubble away the corrosion.
6. To loosen a rusted bolt: applying a cloth soaked in coke –cola to the rusted bolt for several minutes.

7. To bake moist ham: empty a can of coke-cola into the baking pan, wrap the ham in aluminum foil and bake. Thirty minutes before ham is finished, remove the foil allowing the drippings to mix with the coke for sumptuous gravy.
8. To remove grease from clothes empty a can of coke into a load of greasy cloths add detergent and run through a regular cycle the coke-cola will help loosen grease stains it will also clean road haze from your windshield.

F.Y.I. the active ingredient in coke is phosphoric acid. Its Ph. is 2.8 it will dissolve a nail in about 4 days.

To carry coke-cola syrup (the concentrate) the commercial truck must use the Hazardous material place cards reserved for highly corrosive materials. The distributors of coke have been using it to clean the engines of their trucks for years.

STILL WANT TO DRINK IT.

You can't make this stuff up!

Side effects associated with taking stevia:

Stevia is likely to lead to a reduction in blood glucose level.

1. Stevia can cause a reduction in the production of sperm cells as it was in male hamsters given high doses of the plant.
2. It is believed that stevia may cause problems with energy metabolism, especially in children. The plant is capable of blocking carbohydrate absorption, leading to inadequate production or conversion of energy and it shows in the form of fatigue and weakness.
3. Instead of helping in weight loss, stevia may also lead to obesity because it is more than 250 times sweeter than sugar; this tricks the body to overeat since you are not getting any calories from stevia itself. This is more of an indirect side effect of stevia especially when you consume big amounts of stevia over an extended period of time.

4. Another side effect is that it can lead to addiction to sweet things because of the high level of sweetness.
5. Numbness, gas, bloating, nausea and dizziness are some of the other stevia side effects which have been noticed.
6. It is believed that the plant can increase the risk of cancer, though there has not been enough evidence for this, many studies have been carried out to show that if stevia is used excessively, it can lead to D.N.A. mutation, which may lead to cancer, the case of genetic mutation has been seen in animals, and it is not yet clear whether the same thing can happen in humans. This means it is being tested on who I wonder.

There are also different controversies about stevia side effects among pregnant women, and it has been advised that you should not use it to be safe use real sugar or sugar cane. That goes for everyone just cut your quantity in half.

HOLIDAY MENU

THIS COVERS EASTER, THANKSGIVING AND CHRISTMAS

Let's you sit down to dinner feeling comfortable, not uncomfortable. You are able to look before you leap so to speak, knowing that there is nothing on the table that you can't have.

TURKEY AS MUCH AS YOU CAN EAT: WHITE MEAT
GREEN SALAD UNLIMITED
2 TBSP. POTATOES
1 ½ CUPS VETETABLE
1 TSP CRANBERRIES
1 SCOOP OF DRESSING OR 1 SMALL BUN
1 SMALL DESERT YOUR CHOICE
1 FRUIT

My advice to you is that you have a small salad before you go for dinner, it helps with eating the chips and cheese and other fried high fat foods that people put out before dinner.

Go for the dressing instead of the bun as one bun leads to another.

Put on your plate what you are going to eat.

If there happens to be ham as well as turkey and you really want it; have a slice it's up to you if you eat it all. If I said you can't have it, unfortunately it's the only thing you would want.

The fruit should be kept until later on when you are home relaxed after a busy day. It should be a little piece of citrus fruit. Kiwi, pineapple, grapefruit, or orange you choose. Reason for this dinner; will be high fats & high sodium. It doesn't matter who cooks, citrus will help break this down while you sleep.

ENJOY

HOLIDAY CRISIS MANAGEMENT STRATEGY

Away-from home meals and holiday celebrations are unavoidable hazards. They often include traditional foods to satisfy emotional and social- rather than nutritional – needs. Such occasions become excuses for overeating foods we might consider off-limits the rest of the year.

How you deal with these temptations is your choice. Some people try to remain aloof and maintain their strict diet plan, while secretly feeling cheated.

Others abandon their eating plans and give in totally to the celebrations; later regretting the consequences.

Still others manage to maintain a moderate approach, balancing denial and impulse. An event is less likely to be your downfall, however, if you plan a strategy.

Here are some ideas that might help.

1. Be realistic: the eating plan you develop is a road map. Some detours will be beyond your control, while others will be your own doing; accept this fact. Who's to blame is less important than how fast you get back on track.
2. Identify the situations that are most tempting and look for alternatives.

   Food is often used as a catalyst to draw people together. When you give yourself permission to create new reasons for a gathering, you remove some temptation. Ask a friend to join you in a craft class or to view a museum exhibit instead of meeting for lunch. Suggest going to a movie, play or concert instead of a restaurant when you want to celebrate, when eating lunch together is the only practical choice, suggest a restaurant where you know you can eat sensibly. Or propose a picnic where you can bring your own food and perhaps get some exercise. Before holiday celebrations, think about the traditions you most enjoy. How many are related to food? Are some foods prepared because they are expected rather than enjoyed? What's the worst that could happen if some traditional foods were omitted or made in smaller amounts?

3. If you cannot control the situation, remember that you still control what you eat. Serve yourself small helpings and eat slowly. In a restaurant, ask about portion size before ordering. If appropriate; offer to split an order with your companion. If attending a buffet or party, eat a nutritious snack before you go to take the edge off your hunger.
4. Remind yourself why it's important to reach your goal weight. Learn to savour the first bite. Take a small helping and remind yourself that the additional helpings never taste as good as the first.

HOW TO AVOID HOLIDAY HOLD UPS IN YOUR DIET

REVIEW PAST EXPERIENCES

Identify specific instances you will face again

What were the consequences of your past actions?

1. BRAIN STORM ALTERNATIVES

   Write down actions you can take to avoid or resist tempting situations.
2. Practice the desired behaviour
3. Get enough rest. Nothing will sabotage your plans faster than being tired.

Through the years I have worked on different recipes to make them taste good because that's important too. These have been tested by clients, and they got good marks meaning they enjoyed them and used them while losing weight, they are still using them to-day. I hope you enjoy them.

FRESH BERRY TOPPING

Ingredients

1 cup fresh or frozen unsweetened (strawberries, blueberries, raspberries or blackberries)
2 ½ tablespoons honey
½ cup plain yogurt

Directions:

In medium bowl, crush berries and honey. Mix well.
Combine berry mixture with yogurt.

Makes 1 ½ cups = 8 serving

FRUIT CRUMBLE

You can replace the apples in this recipe with peaches, apricots, plums or with two apples and half a cup of cooked rhubarb. If you have a favorite combination, you can use it in this recipe too.

3 large cooking apples, peeled cored and sliced
2 tbsp. water
½ tsp ground cinnamon or 3 cloves

Topping

½ cup rolled oats
2 tbsp. shredded coconut
2 tbsp. mixed fruit
2 tsp chopped nuts
¼ cup bran flakes
¼ cup all-bran

Place apple into a saucepan, add water, and cinnamon or cloves.

Gently simmer for approximately 10 minutes until apple is tender, or microwave, covered on high for 6 minutes.

Lightly grease a small casserole and spoon in apple, remove cloves if used.

Mix toppings ingredients and sprinkle thickly over apple.

Preheat oven to 350%F.

Bake for 30 minutes: or until topping becomes golden.

Serve hot or cold.

To store: cover and refrigerate for up to 4 days

Makes 4 servings
Each serving provides 1 fruit, 1 starch, 1 fat.

Enjoy!

IRISH SODA BREAD

2 cups all- purpose flour
1 teaspoon baking powder
½ teaspoon baking soda
¼ teaspoon salt
3 tablespoons margarine or butter
1 slightly beaten egg white
¾ cup buttermilk
Non-stick spray coating

In a medium bowl stir together flour, baking powder, baking soda and salt. Cut in margarine or butter until mixture resembles coarse crumbs. Make a well in the center of the mixture.

In a small mixing bowl combine egg white and buttermilk. Add all at once to dry mixture. Stir just till moistened.

On a lightly floured surface knead dough 10 to 12 strokes till nearly smooth. Shape into a 7-inch round loaf.

Spray a baking sheet with non-stick spray coating. Place bread sough on baking sheet. With a sharp knife, make 2 slashes on the top to form an X.

Bake in a 375% oven about 30 minutes or till golden brown.

Serve warm.

Makes 1 loaf = 16 servings
Each serving provides 1 starch, ½ fat.

Enjoy!

BLUEBERRY GEMS

1 ½ cups, all-purpose flour
¼ cup sugar
1 ½ teaspoons baking powder
¼ teaspoon salt
2 egg whites
2/3 cup orange juice
2 tablespoons cooking oil
1 teaspoon vanilla
1 cup fresh or frozen blueberries
Non-stick spray coating

In a medium mixing bowl combine flour, sugar, baking powder and salt. In a small mixing bowl beat egg whites, orange juice, oil and vanilla. Add to dry ingredients, stirring just until moistened. Fold in blueberries.

Spray muffin cups*with non-stick spray coating. Fill muffin cups half full.

Bake in a 400% oven about 17 minutes or until golden
Cool slightly before serving.
Makes 36 muffins

Each serving provides= 1 starch, ¼ fat, ¼ fruit
Serving = 2 muffins

Enjoy!

BAKED CUSTARD

Can be served hot or cold

2 eggs
¼ cup sugar
1 tsp vanilla extract
Sprinkling of ground nutmeg

In a bowl, lightly beat the eggs

Gradually add the milk to the egg mixture, stirring constantly. Stir in the vanilla extract and sugar.

Pour mixture into a pie or soufflé dish or dishes. Sprinkle with nutmeg.

Stand the baking dish or dishes in a large baking dish. Carefully pour enough water into the large baking dish to reach two thirds up the outside of the pie or soufflé dish.

Preheat oven to 350% F

Bake for 35 minutes if you are using individual dishes, 45 minutes if you are using one big dish. The custard should be lightly browned and set in the center.

Makes 4 servings
Each serving provides = ½ protein.

ENJOY!

LEMON AND CINNAMON CHEESECAKE

You must make this recipe the day before you want to serve it to allow the filling to set.

Crust

1 cup shredded whole wheat cracker crumbs
2oz almonds, crushed
1 tbsp. margarine, melted
2 tsp water
2 tsp cinnamon

Filling

10oz buttermilk
8oz ricotta cheese
Juice of 2 lemons
Zest of 1 lemon
1 tsp vanilla extract
1 tbsp. sugar
1 tbsp. powdered gelatin
2 tbsp. water

Garnish

Kiwi & strawberries (optional)
2 tsp cinnamon
Instructions
Combine all ingredients for biscuit base
Press mixture into lined pie dish and refrigerate for 30 minutes

Filling

Mix buttermilk with ricotta cheese, lemon juice, lemon zest, vanilla extract and sugar. Beat until smooth and fluffy.

Dissolve gelatin in hot water. Cool slightly and fold into buttermilk mixture and blend well

Pour into pie base and refrigerate until set

Next day, decorate with sliced kiwi or strawberries and a sprinkle of cinnamon.

To store cover and refrigerate for up to three days

Makes 8 servings: each serving provides = 1 protein, 1 starch, 1 fat.

ENJOY!

CINNAMON ROLLS WITH ORANGE GLAZE

1-pound, loaf frozen bread sough, thawed
1 tbsp. margarine melted
1 tbsp. sugar
1 teaspoon ground cinnamon
Non-stick spray coating
½ cup powdered sugar
¼ teaspoon finely shredded orange peel
2 to 3 teaspoons orange juice

On a floured surface, roll dough into a 12+8 inch rectangle; (if the dough is difficult to roll out, let it rest for a short time and roll again. Repeat as necessary). Brush dough with melted margarine; sprinkle evenly with the 1 tbsp. sugar and cinnamon.

Roll up dough, beginning from one of the long sides. Seal seam slice into 12 one inch pieces.

Spray coating, place rolls in pan with one cut side down. Cover and let rise in a warm place till nearly double; about 30 minutes.

Bake in a 375% oven for 20 to 25 minutes or till lightly browned. Cool slightly; remove from pan.

For glaze; in a small bowl stir together powdered sugar, and orange peel, and enough orange juice to make desired consistency. Drizzle over warm rolls.

Serve warm.

Makes 12 servings
Each serving provides = 1 starch & ¼ fat

ENJOY!

PUMPKIN PIE

Pastry

2 tbsp. margarine
1 cup whole wheat flour
1 egg yolk
Juice of ½ lemon plus cold water to make 1/3 cup

Filling

2 cups firm pumpkin puree
¼ cup ricotta cheese
¼ cup plain yogurt
½ cup milk
2 eggs, separated
½ tsp nutmeg
1 tsp cinnamon
¼ tsp ginger
¼ tsp ground cloves
Juice and zest of 1 lemon
Sugar to taste

Garnish

Ground cinnamon
Pastry: Preheat oven to 350%F
Rub margarine into flour until mixture resembles fine bread crumbs
Mix egg yolk with juice and water
Mix liquid into flour with a knife, to make soft dough
Turn out onto a floured board. Knead lightly, leave for 15 minutes

Roll out on floured board, cover base and sides of pie dish with pastry. Add a second strip around top-edge and pinch as a decorative edge. Prick pastry with a fork and place in oven, bake until lightly browned.

Filling

Combine in a bowl pumpkin, ricotta, yogurt, and milk and egg yolks. Beat well

Add spices, lemon juice, zest and sweetener. Check taste and adjust if necessary. Beat egg whites until soft peaks form, fold into pumpkin mixture.

Pour into pastry shell and bake in preheated oven until set (about 1 hour)

Sprinkle with a little cinnamon to serve.

To store: cover and refrigerate for up to two days

Makes 6 serving

Each serving provides = ¾ protein, 1 fat, 1 starch, 1/3 fruit. ENJOY!

CARROT PINEAPPLE ZUCCJINI LOAF

Preheat oven to 350%F spray 9+5 inch loaf pan with pam

¼ cup margarine
1 cup sugar
1 egg
1 egg white
2 tsp cinnamon
1 ½ tsp vanilla
¼ tsp nutmeg
¾ cup grated carrot
¾ cup grated zucchini
½ cup drained crushed pineapple
1/3 cup raisins
1 ¼ cups, all- purpose flour
½ cup whole wheat flour
1 tsp baking powder
1 tsp baking soda

In a large bowl or food processor, cream margarine with sugar.

Add egg, and egg white, cinnamon, vanilla and nutmeg; beat well.

Stir in carrot, zucchini, pineapple and raisins, blend until well combined.

Combine all purpose and whole wheat flours, baking powder and baking soda. Add to bowl and mix just until combined.

Pour into loaf pan, and bake for 35 to 45 minutes or until tester inserted into centre comes out dry.

Makes 20 slices
Each serving provides = 1 starch, 1 fat, ½ vegetable and ½ fruit.

ENJOY!

CARROT –PINEAPPLE LOAF

Preheat oven to 350%F

Ingredients

1-3/4 cups all-purpose flour
2 teaspoons baking powder
1 teaspoon each baking soda & ground cinnamon
¼ teaspoon each salt & ground nutmeg
1 cup packed brown sugar
¼ cup each canola oil & pineapple juice
1 egg
1 egg white
1 teaspoon vanilla
¾ cup shredded carrots
8oz drained crushed pineapple

Combine flour, baking powder, baking soda, cinnamon, salt and nutmeg in a large bowl, stir well and set aside.

In a small bowl, whisk together brown sugar, oil, pineapple juice, egg, egg white and vanilla.

Add to flour mixture, mix until dry ingredients are moistened. Stir in carrots & pineapple. Batter will be thick.

Spray an 8+4 –inch loaf pan with non-stick spray: Spoon batter into pan.

Bake for 40-50 minutes or until wooden pick inserted in center comes out clean.

Cool on wire rack.

Makes 1 loaf: 12 slices
Each serving provides = 1 starch, 1 fat, ¼ fruit

ENJOY!

BANANA NUT RAISIN LOAF

Preheat oven to 375%F. spray 9+5- inch loaf pan with pam

Ingredients

2 large ripe bananas
1/3 cup soft margarine
½ cup sugar
1 egg
1egg white
¼ cup hot water
1 1/3 cups whole wheat flour
¾ tsp baking soda
¼ cup raisins
1/3 cup chopped pecans or walnuts

In bowl or food processor, beat bananas and margarine, beat in sugar, egg, egg white and water until smooth.

Combine flour and baking soda, stir into batter along with raisins and all but a few of the pecans or walnuts, mix until blended. Do not over-mix. Pour into pan; arrange reserved nuts down middle of mixture.

Bake for 35 to 45 minutes or until tester inserted into centre comes out dry.

Makes 10 slices
Each serving provides = 1 starch and 1 fat

ENJOY!

SOUR CREAM APPLE PIE

Preheat oven to 350%

Ingredients

5 ½ cups sliced peeled apples (5 to 6 apples)
½ cup sugar
½ cup plain yogurt
½ cup sour cream
¼ cup raisins
2 tbsp. all- purpose flour
1 tsp cinnamon
1 egg, lightly beaten
1 tsp vanilla

Crust

1 ½ cups graham wafer crumbs
2 tbsp. margarine, melted
1 tbsp. brown sugar
1 tbsp. water

Topping

¼ cup brown sugar
3 tbsp. all-purpose flour
2 tbsp. rolled oats
½ tsp cinnamon
1 tbsp. margarine

Crust: in a bowl, combine graham crumbs, margarine, sugar and water; pat onto bottom and sides of pan. Refrigerate.

In large bowl, combine apples, sugar, yogurt, sour cream, raisins, flour, cinnamon, egg, and vanilla; toss together until well mixed. Pour over crust.

Topping: in a small bowl, combine sugar, flour, rolled oats and cinnamon; cut in margarine until crumbly, sprinkle over pie; bake for 30 to 40 minutes or until topping is browned and apples are tender.

Makes 16 slices each serving = 1 slice
Serving provides = 1 starch, 1 fat, 1 fruit

ENJOY!

LEMON POPPY SEED LOAF

Preheat oven to 350%F. Spray 9+5 inch loaf pan

Ingredients

¾ cup sugar
1/3 cup margarine
1 egg
2 tsp grated lemon rind
3 tbsp. lemon juice
1/3 cup milk
1 ¼ cups all-purpose flour
1 tbsp. poppy seeds
1 tsp baking powder
½ tsp baking soda
1/3 cup plain yogurt

Glaze

¼ cup icing sugar
2 tbsp. lemon juice

In a large bowl, beat together sugar, margarine, egg, lemon rind and juice, mixing well. Add milk, mixing well.

Combine flour, poppy seeds, baking powder and baking soda; add to bowl alternately with yogurt, mixing just until incorporated. Do not over mix.

Pour into pan; and bake for 35-40 minutes or until tester inserted into centre comes out dry.

Glaze: prick holes in top of loaf with fork. Combine icing sugar with lemon juice; pour over loaf.

Makes 10 servings =1 slice

Each serving provides 1 starch 1 fat

ENJOY!

FRUITY BAKED RICE PUDDING

Preheat oven to: 350%F

3 ½ cups milk
5 tbsp. uncooked brown or white rice
1 tbsp. sugar
4 tbsp. raisins
4 tbsp. dried peaches or apricots

Garnish:

Ground cinnamon or nutmeg

Combine milk, rice and sugar, and place mixture in baking dish
Cover and bake for 45 minutes
Remove from oven, add dried fruit and stir
Leave uncovered and return to oven. Cook for another 45 to 60 minutes until rice is cooked. A skin will form on top of rice.
Serve hot or cold, garnish with ground cinnamon or nutmeg
To store: cover and refrigerate for up to three days.

Makes 4 servings
Each serving provides = 1 fruit, ½ starch

ENJOY!

BANANA BREAD

Preheat oven to 350%F

Ingredients

1 ½ cups all-purpose flour
1 ¼ teaspoons baking powder
½ teaspoon baking soda
½ teaspoon ground cinnamon
1/8 teaspoon sea salt
2 slightly beaten egg whites
1 cup mashed banana
¾ cup sugar
¼ cup cooking oil

In a medium mixing bowl stir together flour, baking powder, baking soda, cinnamon and sea salt.

In a large mixing bowl stir together egg whites, banana, sugar and oil

Stir flour mixture into banana mixture just till moistened

Spray an 8+4+2 inch loaf pan with non-stick spray coating. Spread batter in prepared pan. Bake for 45 to 50 minutes or a toothpick inserted near center comes out clean.

Cool bread in pan for 10 minutes. Remove from pan and cool thoroughly on a wire rack. For easier slicing, wrap bread in plastic wrap and store overnight.

Makes 1 loaf = 16 servings
Each serving provides = 1 starch, 1 fat

Enjoy!

BROWNIE BITES

Ingredients

2 tbsp. margarine
1/3 cup sugar
¼ cup cold water
½ tsp vanilla
½ cup all-purpose flour
2 tbsp. cocoa powder
½ tsp baking powder
2 tbsp. finely chopped walnuts or pecans
Non-stick spray coating
1 tsp. powdered sugar

Directions:

In a small saucepan melt margarine; remove from heat stir in sugar, vanilla and water. Stir in flour, cocoa powder and baking powder until well mixed. Stir in chopped nuts.

Spray the bottom only of an 8+4+2 – inch loaf pan with non-stick coating.

Pour batter into pan.

Bake in a 350%F. oven about 20 minutes or until a toothpick inserted near the center comes out clean.

Cool thoroughly. Remove cake from pan.

Cut into 8 bars. Sprinkle with powdered sugar.

Makes 8 servings
Each serving provides = 1 starch, 1 fat

Enjoy

FANTASY CAKE

Ingredients

1 ¾ cups; all - purpose flour
1 cup; granulated sugar
½ cup; unpacked brown sugar
1 tsp baking powder
1 tsp baking soda
1 cup crushed pineapple in juice
1/3 cup mashed banana (ripe)
3 eggs
¾ tsp vanilla
½ cup mini chocolate chips
1/3 cup chopped walnuts
1 tbsp. all-purpose flour

Preheat oven to 350%F.

Directions:

Combine flour, sugar, brown sugar, baking powder and baking soda in a medium bowl. Mix well and set aside.

In a large bowl, blend together crushed pineapple and juice, banana, eggs and vanilla using electric mixer on low- speed. Do not overbeat. Gradually add flour mixture and beat on medium-high speed until all flour has been incorporated.

In a small bowl, mix together chocolate chips, walnuts and 1 tbsp. flour. Fold into batter.

Spray an 8+8 – inch baking pan with non-stick spray. Pour batter into pan.

Bake for 40 to 45 minutes until wooden pick inserted in center comes out clean.

Let cool completely in pan. Cut into 12 pieces and store at room temperature in an airtight container.

Makes 12 servings
Each serving provides = 1 starch, ¼ fruit, ¼ fat, ¼ protein

Enjoy!

ORANGE- GLAZED COFFEE CAKE

Ingredients

¼ cup soft margarine
1 cup granulated sugar
3 eggs
1 ½ cups orange juice
1 ½ tsp grated orange rind
1 cup whole wheat flour
1 cup all-purpose flour
1 tsp cinnamon
1 tsp baking soda
1 tsp baking powder

GLAZE

½ cup icing sugar
4 tsp frozen orange concentrate, thawed

Preheat oven to 350%F.
9- Inch (3L) Bundt pan sprayed with non-stick vegetable spray

Directions:

In large bowl or food processor, cream together margarine and sugar. Beat in eggs, orange juice and rind until well blended.

Combine whole wheat and all- purpose flours, cinnamon, baking powder and baking soda, add to creamed mixture and mix until well blended. Pour into pan. Bake for 35 to 40 minutes or until cake tester comes out clean. Let cool.

Glaze: Mix icing sugar with orange juice concentrate; pour over cake, allow icing to drip down sides.

Makes 16 slices
Each serving provides = 1 starch, 1 fat
You can serve this cake without the glaze.
Bake a day before, or freeze for up to six weeks.

Enjoy!

FRUIT CRUMBLE

You can replace the apples in this recipe with peaches, apricots or plumbs or with two apples and half a cup of cooked rhubarb. If you have a favorite combination, you can use it in this recipe too.

Ingredients

3 large cooking apples, peeled cored and sliced
2 tbsp. water
½ tsp ground cinnamon or 3 cloves

Topping:

½ cup rolled oats
2 tbsp. shredded coconut
2 tbsp. mixed fruit
2 tsp chopped nuts
¼ cup bran flakes
¼ cup all-bran

Directions:

Place apples into a saucepan; add water and cinnamon or cloves.

Gently simmer for approximately 10 minutes until apple is tender, or microwave, covered on high for 6 minutes.

Lightly grease a small casserole and spoon apple, removing cloves if used.

Mix topping ingredients and sprinkle thickly over apples.

Preheat oven to 350%F.

Bake for 30 minutes or until; topping becomes golden.

Serve hot or cold

To store: cover and refrigerate for up to four days.

Makes 4 servings
Each serving provides = 1 fruit, 1 starch, 1 fat

Enjoy!

BANANA BREAD

Ingredients

2 cups all-purpose flour
¾ cup whole wheat flour
1 cup unpacked brown sugar
1 ½ tsp baking powder
½ tsp baking soda
1 tsp ground cinnamon
½ tsp sea salt
3 eggs
2 tbsp. margarine, melted
¾ cup plain yogurt
1 tsp vanilla
2 cups mashed ripe bananas
½ cup chopped walnuts

Preheat oven to 325%F.

Directions:

Combine flours and next five ingredients in a large bowl. Set aside.

In a medium bowl, beat eggs, margarine, yogurt and vanilla with a whisk until smooth. Add bananas and whisk again.

Add banana mixture to flour mixture. Stir until dry ingredients are moistened. Stir in walnuts.

Spray a 9+5- inch loaf pan with non-stick spray.

Pour batter into pan. Bake for 1 hour and 20 minutes, or until toothpick inserted in center comes out clean. Remove from pan and let cool.

Makes 1 large loaf = 16 servings
Each serving provides = 1 starch, ½ fruit, ¼ protein

Enjoy!

HOT JAMAICAN PINEAPPLE

Ingredients

½ medium pineapple; cut lengthwise with top intact
3 bananas, peeled and chopped
4 tsp brown sugar
¼ cup shredded coconut

Directions:

Preheat oven to 350%F

Cut pineapple out of skin, being careful not to pierce skin.

Scoop out any remaining pulp and juice and retain.

Chop pineapple into chunks, discarding core. Add to pulp and juice in bowl.

Add bananas and brown sugar.

Spoon fruit and juices into shell and sprinkle with coconut

Place in baking dish, and bake for 30-45 minutes until fruit is heated through and coconut is toasted.

Spoon: into serving dishes.

Makes 4 servings
Each serving provides = 1 fruit, ½ fat

Enjoy!

CHOCOLATE SHAKES

Ingredients

4 cups cold milk
1 package instant chocolate pudding mix (4 serving size)
Few drops mint or rum extract (optional)
½ cup ice cubes

In a blender combine milk, pudding mix and mint or rum extract, if desired

Cover and blend until smooth, add ice cubes; cover and blend till combined. Let stand 3 minutes to thicken slightly

Makes 5 eight ounce servings

Enjoy

CHOCOLATE MINT CAKE

Ingredients

½ cup firmly packed cocoa powder
½ cup very hot strong coffee
1 tsp pure vanilla extract
2 eggs, separated
½ cup granulated sugar
2 egg whites
¾ tsp mint extract
½ cup cake flour, sifted
Pinch salt
2 tsp powdered sugar
8 sprigs mint (optional)

Directions: Preheat oven to 350%F.

Line bottom of an 8-inch round cake pan with parchment paper or non-stick oven liner film, spray liner and sides of pan with butter- flavored non-stick cooking spray. Place cocoa powder, hot coffee and vanilla in a medium sized bowl. Whisk to dissolve cocoa. Set aside to cool. Combine 2 egg yolks and ¼ cup of the granulated sugar in the top of a double boiler or in a small saucepan placed in a skillet half filled with water. Heat bottom pan of water to a simmer, and whisk the egg and sugar mixture just until the mixture thickens and the sugar crystals are dissolved. (Do not overheat, or you will make sweet scrambled eggs).Transfer the yolk mixture to the bowl of a mixer. Beat mixture until it is the consistency of a light frosting and has doubled in volume. Gently fold this into the chocolate mixture with a spatula. Place 4 egg whites in a dry, grease free mixing bowl. Beat whites until soft peaks form. Very gradually add the remaining ¼ cup granulated sugar and mint extract, beating the meringue until stiff peaks form. Sift cake flour and salt onto chocolate mixture. Fold flour into chocolate with a rubber spatula until no flour shows. Transfer half of the chocolate mixture to the bowl of meringue. Fold it in very gently. Repeat process with remainder of chocolate. Turn the mixture into the prepared pan; use a spatula to level the top. Put pan on middle rack of oven; bake about 20 minute until cake is puffed but springs back to the touch or an inserted toothpick comes out clean. Remove from oven; cool 5 to 10 minutes on wire rack. Put rack on top of cake. Invert to remove cake from pan. Cool cake completely. When ready to serve. Sift powdered sugar over cake. Garnish each piece with a sprig of mint if desired. Makes 8 servings = 1/8 of cake = 1 starch

WHIPPED TOPPING

Ingredients
1/3 cup milk
1/3 cup dry milk solids
1-2 tsp honey to taste
¼ tsp vanilla

Directions:

Pour milk into a small metal mixing bowl. Set bowl in freezer until ice crystals begin to form, about 15 -20 minutes. Chill beaters from mixer in freezer as well.

Using a hand held electric mixer, beat dry milk solids into milk. Continue to beat on high until soft peaks form about 2 minutes. Add honey to taste and vanilla beat until stiff peaks form; about 2 additional minutes. Use within 20 minutes to avoid cream separating.

Prep time 8 minutes: chilling time 20 minutes
Makes 6 servings= ¼ cup

Enjoy!

RASPBERRY CHEESECAKE

Ingredients

1 package unsweetened raspberry
1 container yogurt
2 tbsp. sugar
2 packages vanilla or strawberry pudding (use ½ the milk of package directions)
Mix together. Pour mixture over graham cracker
Refrigerate for 2 hours

Each serving provides = ¼ protein, ½ fat, ¼ starch, ¼ fruit

Enjoy!

TROPICAL PUNCH

Ingredients

2 cups water
¼ cup sugar
1 inch piece of fresh gingerroot or a 3 inch stick of cinnamon
6oz can frozen pineapple or orange juice concentrate
1/3 cup lime juice
2 cups carbonated water chilled
Ice
4 lime slices, halved

Directions:

In a medium saucepan combine water, sugar and gingerroot or cinnamon.
Bring to a boil; reduce heat, cover and simmer for 10 minutes.
Remove from heat. Remove and discard gingerroot or cinnamon stick.
Stir in pineapple or orange juice.
Pour into a pitcher cover and chill for 4 hours.
Just before serving stir in carbonated water. Serve over ice.
Garnish with lime slices.

Makes 8- (5 ounce servings)

Enjoy!

TOMATO SOUP

Ingredients

½ cup chopped onion
¾ cup chopped green or sweet red pepper
1 tbsp. margarine
1 ½ teaspoon fresh snipped basil or ½ teaspoon dried basil crushed
1/8 teaspoon ground red pepper (optional)
2 cups tomato juice
1 cup buttermilk
Fresh basil leaves or lime slices (optional)

In a small saucepan; cook onion and green or sweet red pepper in margarine till very tender. Stir in basil and ground red pepper, if desired. Cook and stir for 1 minute more.

Remove from heat

In a blender container combine cooked vegetable mixture, tomato juice, and buttermilk. Cover and blend till smooth.

Return mixture to saucepan and heat through. Or chill thoroughly.

Garnish each serving with fresh basil leaves or lime slices, if desired.

Makes 4 servings
Each serving provides = 1 vegetable, ¼ fat

Enjoy!

FRESH TOMATO DILL SOUP

Ingredients

1 celery stalk, chopped
1 tbsp. olive oil
1 tsp crushed garlic
1 med carrot, chopped
1 cup chopped, onion
2 cups chicken stock
5 cups chopped ripe tomatoes
3 tbsp. tomato paste
2 tsp sugar
3 tbsp. chopped fresh dill

In large non-stick saucepan, heat oil sauté garlic, carrot, celery and onion until softened, approximately 5 minutes.

Add stock, tomatoes and tomato paste, reduce heat, cover and simmer for 20 minutes stirring occasionally.

Puree in food processor until smooth, add sugar and dill; mix well

Makes 6 servings =1 cup
Each serving provides = 1 veg

Enjoy!

ASPARAGUS AND LEEK SOUP

Ingredients

¾ lb asparagus
1 ½ tsp vegetable oil
1 tsp crushed garlic
1 cup chopped onion
2 leeks, sliced
3 ½ cups chicken stock
1 cup diced potato
Sea salt and pepper

Trim asparagus; cut stalks into pieces and set aside

In large non-stick saucepan, heat oil; sauté garlic, onion leeks and asparagus stalks just until softened approximately 10 minutes

Add stock and potato; reduce heat, cover and simmer for 20 to 25 minutes or until vegetables are tender. Puree in food processor until smooth. Taste and adjust seasoning with sea salt and pepper. Return to saucepan.

Steam or microwave reserved asparagus tips just until tender; add to soup; and serve. This soup can be served hot or cold.

Makes 4 to 6 servings
Each serving provides = ½ vegetable, ¼ starch, ¼ fat

Enjoy!

GREEN PEA, SPINACH AND CHICKEN SOUP

Ingredients

2 cups frozen peas
3 cups chicken stock
8oz packet frozen spinach
1 cup chopped cooked chicken
2 tsp curry powder

Cook peas in stock until tender (approximately 15 minutes)

Combine in food processor until partly broken down and return to saucepan.

Add spinach and simmer until the spinach is thoroughly heated (approximately 10 minutes) add chicken and curry powder; and bring to a boil and serve.

To store: cover and refrigerate for up to two days

Makes 4 servings
Each serving provides = 1 vegetable ½ protein

Enjoy!

CHEESE AND VEGETABLE SOUP

Ingredients

1cup chicken broth
½ cup chopped peeled potato
¼ cup chopped celery
¼ cup chopped carrot
¼ cup chopped green or sweet red pepper
1 cup milk
2 tbsp. all-purpose flour
¼ cup shredded cheese
Dash ground nutmeg

In medium saucepan combine chicken broth, potato, celery, carrot and green or sweet red pepper. Bring to a boil; reduce heat. Cover and simmer for 10 to 12 minutes until vegetables are tender. In a small bowl stir together milk and flour; stir into saucepan. Cook and stir till thickened and bubbly. Cook and stir for 1 minute more. Stir in cheese till melted; stir in nutmeg.

Makes 4 servings
Each serving provides = 1 vegetable ¼ protein ¼ starch and ¼ fat

Enjoy!

PORK AND VEGETABLE NOODLE SOUP

Ingredients

7oz soup bones
4 cups water
8oz pork fillet, diced
1 medium carrot, grated
2 sticks celery, chopped
½ parsnip, grated
½ turnip, grated
1 medium leek, chopped
2 tbsp. chopped parsley
½ tsp black pepper
3oz noodles

Garnish: shallots, chopped

Place soup bones and water in saucepan and bring to boil. Simmer for 1 hour
Strain and discard bones
Heat saucepan and fry pork fillet until browned
Add pork, carrot, celery, parsnip, turnip, leek, and black pepper to stock
Cook until meat and vegetables are tender
Add noodles and cook for 5 to 10 minutes or until noodles are tender
Spoon into individual bowls, garnish with chopped shallots

Makes 4 servings
Each serving provides = 1 protein, ¾ vegetable, ¾ starch

Enjoy!

CAULIFLOWER POTATO SOUP

Ingredients

1 tbsp. vegetable oil
1 tsp crushed garlic
1 cup chopped onions
1 medium cauliflower (separated into florets)
4 cups chicken stock
2 small potatoes, peeled and chopped
2 tbsp. chopped fresh chives

In large non-stick saucepan, heat oil; sauté garlic and onions until softened, approximately 5 minutes. Add cauliflower, stock and potatoes; bring to a boil. Cover, reduce heat and simmer for 25 minutes or until tender. Transfer to food processor and puree until creamy and smooth. Return to saucepan and thin with more stock if desired. Ladle into bowls; sprinkle with chives.

Makes 4 servings
Each serving provides = 1 veg ½ starch ¼fat

Enjoy!

BROCCOLI AND SWEET CORN SOUP

Ingredients

1 large head of broccoli
2 cups chicken stock
15oz can creamed sweet corn
1 stick celery, finely chopped
6 shallots, finely sliced
½ tsp sea salt (optional) pepper to taste
Garnish: chopped chives

Break broccoli into florets and cook it in stock until tender (approximately 10 minutes). Blend until smooth in food processor. Add creamed sweet corn, celery, shallots and seasonings. Reheat and serve, garnished with chopped chives. To store: cover and refrigerate for up to three days.

Makes 4 servings
Each serving provides 1 starch, 2 vegetables, and ½ fat

Enjoy!

BEEF AND BEAN SOUP

Ingredients

8oz lean ground beef
1 medium onion, diced
1 small clove garlic, diced
2 sticks celery, diced
14oz can tomatoes
1 tbsp. tomato paste
3 cups water
½ tsp oregano, dried or 1 tsp fresh
½ tsp paprika
½ tsp ground cumin
2 tsp white vinegar
15oz can kidney beans, drained and rinsed

Fry meat, add onion and garlic and cook until juices evaporate and ground beef is well browned; add celery, tomatoes, tomato paste, water, oregano, paprika, cumin and vinegar. Bring to a boil. Add beans and reduce heat to low, cover and simmer for 30 minutes.

To store: cover and refrigerate for up to three days

Makes 5-6 servings
Each serving provides = 1 protein, 1 ½ vegetables ½ starch

Enjoy!

GREEN PEA, SPINACH, AND CHICKEN SOUP

Ingredients

2 cups frozen peas
3 cups chicken stock
8oz package frozen spinach
1 cup chopped cooked chicken
2 tsp curry powder

Cook peas in stock until tender (approximately 15 minutes). Combine in food processor until partly broken down and return to saucepan, add spinach and simmer until the spinach is thoroughly heated (approximately 10 minutes). Add chicken and curry powder; bring to a boil and serve.

To store: cover and refrigerate for up to two days.

Makes 4 servings
Each serving provides = 1 vegetable ½ protein. Enjoy!

VEGETABLE AND BEAN MINESTRONE SOUP

Ingredients

1 tbsp. vegetable oil
1 tsp crushed garlic
1 ½ cups finely chopped onion
1 medium carrot, finely chopped
1 small celery stalk, finely chopped
4 ½ cups beef or chicken stock
1 ½ cups finely chopped peeled potato
1 ½ cups chopped broccoli
1 can 19oz tomatoes, crushed
¾ cup cooked chick peas
2 bay leaves
1 ½ tsp each dried basil and oregano
Pepper
1/3 cup broken spaghetti

In large non-stick saucepan, heat oil; sauté` garlic, onion, carrot and celery until softened, approximately 5 minutes.

Add stock, potatoes, broccoli, tomatoes, chick peas, bay leaves, basil and oregano; cover and simmer for approximately 40 minutes or until vegetables are tender, stirring occasionally. Remove bay leaves. Season with pepper

Add pasta; cook for 10 minutes, stirring often or until spaghetti is firm to the bite.

Makes 6 servings
Each serving provides = 1 vegetable ½ starch ¼ fat ¼ proteins

Enjoy!

GARDEN VEGETABLE SOUP

Ingredients

1 cup chopped leek, white portion only, thoroughly washed
2 celery stalks with leaves, chopped
¾ cup chopped onion
1 cup diced carrots
2 cloves garlic, chopped
¼ cup water+3 cups of water or (vegetable stock)
1 ¼ cups tomato juice (no salt if available)
1 cup diced potato
1 cup cauliflower florets
¼ cup chopped fresh parsley or 2 tablespoons dried
1 teaspoon dried basil
1 teaspoon Italian seasoning blend
1/8 teaspoon white pepper (optional)
1 ½ teaspoons honey
1 cup chopped greens
Fresh lemon wedges

Combine leek, celery, onion, carrots, garlic and ¼ cup water in soup pot.

Cover and cook over med heat 5 minutes stirring occasionally.

Add 3 cups of water, tomato juice, potato, cauliflower, parsley and herbs; bring to a boil, cover, reduce heat and simmer 30 minutes until vegetables are tender.

Add honey and greens. Cover and cook 5 minutes longer, or until greens are wilted.

Serve with lemon wedges perched on the rim of each bowl so the fresh lemon can be squeezed in to taste at the table.

Makes 6 servings
Each serving provides= 1 vegetable ¼ starch

Enjoy!

FRENCH ONION SOUP

Ingredients

2 large yellow onions sliced into rings
1 clove garlic, minced
2 cups chicken stock
2 cups beef stock
½ cup unsweetened apple juice
1 teaspoon each, Worcestershire sauce and ground thyme
½ teaspoon ground rosemary
4 slices French stick bread
2 cloves garlic, peeled and halved
1/3 cup shredded mozzarella cheese (about 1 ½ ounces)
Fresh parsley for garnish

Combine onions, garlic, and ¼ cup of chicken stock in a large saucepan. Cook over medium –low heat for 25 minutes. Onions should be tender and golden brown. Add remaining chicken stock, beef stock, apple juice, Worcestershire sauce, thyme and rosemary. Bring to a boil. Reduce heat to low, cover and simmer for 15 minutes.

Meanwhile, toast bread slices under broiler for 1-2 min on each side. Be careful not to burn them. Remove from oven and rub each piece of toasted bread with the cut sides of the garlic halves (keep broiler on).

Ladle soup into 4 oven proof bowls. Place toasted bread slices in each bowl and top with shredded cheese. Broil until cheese is melted. Garnish with fresh parsley. Serve immediately.

Makes 4 servings
Each serving provides = 1 starch ½ fat ¼ vegetable

Enjoy!

MINESTRONE SOUP

Ingredients

2 medium onions
2 medium carrots
2 sticks celery
½ bell- pepper
2 medium potatoes
4oz green beans, sliced
1 cup shredded cabbage
4 large tomatoes
2 tsp olive oil
1 cup dried cannellini beans
4 cups water
3 bay leaves
½ tsp sea salt
¼ tsp pepper
Juice of ½ lemon
1 tsp dried mixed herbs or two tsp mixed herbs

Peel and chop vegetables
Heat oil in saucepan
Add onions and cook until lightly browned.
Add carrots, celery, bell pepper and potatoes. Cook until lightly colored
Now add green beans, cabbage and tomatoes. Cook until just tender
Add dried beans, water, herbs and lemon juice
Simmer with lid on until beans are tender (approximately 1 hour)
Check for flavor and adjust to taste.

To store: cover and refrigerate for up to three days

Makes 4-6 servings
Each serving provides= 1 vegetable 1 starch 1 protein ½ fat

ENJOY!

HUNGARIAN SOUP

Ingredients

3 cups chicken stock
1 cup finely shredded red cabbage
3 small onions thinly sliced
1 clove garlic, crushed
2 large tomatoes, peeled and quartered
1 large apple, peeled and chopped
Coarsely, ground black pepper, to taste
¼ tsp ground all spice
Garnish: chives

Place stock in a large saucepan and bring to a boil
Add all other ingredients
Cover and simmer for 30 minutes
Serve, garnished with a sprinkling of chopped chives
To store: cover and refrigerate for up to three days
Makes 4 servings

Each serving provides = 1 vegetable ¼ fruit

Enjoy!

HOT AND SOUR SOUP

Ingredients

3 chicken breast fillets (1lb)
2 ½ tbsp. white vinegar
2 tsp olive oil
4oz firm tofu
4 cups chicken stock
½ medium red bell pepper, cut into thin strips
4oz mushrooms
4oz can bamboo shoots, drained and rinsed
4 shallots, chopped
2 tbsp. cornstarch
1 egg

With a sharp knife, slice chicken very finely
Place chicken slices in bowl with vinegar
Place oil in heavy saucepan and heat on high. Add tofu and stir- fry until tender about 3 minutes. Remove from saucepan.

Pour chicken stock into saucepan with bell peppers, mushrooms, bamboo shoots and shallots; heat to boiling: cover and simmer 10 minutes or until vegetables are tender; add chicken and tofu, heat to boiling. Mix cornstarch and a small amount of water in a separate bowl; slowly stir cornstarch mixture into boiling soup; cook, stirring constantly, until slightly thickened. Remove from heat. Beat egg in a small bowl; then slowly pour egg mixture into soup, stirring quickly until egg swirls and has just set. Spoon soup into individual bowls.

To store: cover and refrigerate for up to three days

Makes 4-6 servings
Each serving provides = 1 protein 1vegetable 1 fat

ENJOY!

CREAMY CARROT SOUP

Ingredients

4 cups chicken stock
1 cup coarsely chopped onions
2 cloves garlic, minced
2 tsp grated ginger root
3 cups coarsely chopped carrots
1 tsp ground thyme
½ cup orange juice
½ cup buttermilk
3-4 drops hot pepper sauce
¼ tsp black pepper
1 tbsp. chopped fresh parsley

Pour ½ cup of the chicken stock in a large saucepan. Add onions, garlic, and ginger root. Cook over medium-high heat for 3 minutes. Stir in remaining broth, carrots, thyme and orange juice. Bring to a boil. Reduce heat to medium-low. Cover and boil gently for 20 minutes, or until carrots are tender.

Work in batches, transfer soup to a blender and process until smooth. Return to saucepan. Reduce heat to low. Stir in buttermilk, hot pepper sauce and pepper. Do not let soup boil. Stir until heated through, about 12 minutes.

Ladle into serving bowls and sprinkle with chopped fresh parsley.

Makes 6 servings
Each serving provides= 1 vegetable

ENJOY!

CHICKPEA SOUP

Ingredients

4 cups chicken stock
1 can: 28oz chick-pea's, drained and rinsed
3 cups peeled, cubed potatoes
1 ½ cups thinly sliced carrots
½ cup each chopped onions and chopped celery
1 tbsp. lemon juice
1 bay leaf
1 clove garlic, minced
½ tsp each ground sage and ground thyme
¼ tsp each black pepper and sea salt
½ cup chopped fresh parsley

Combine all ingredients except parsley in a large saucepan. Bring to a boil. Reduce heat to med – low. Cover and simmer for 20 minutes.

Using a potato masher, mash vegetables until soup resembles a coarsely pureed mixture. Stir in parsley and serve.

Makes 6 servings
Each serving provides = ½ protein ½ vegetable ½ fat

ENJOY!

CURRIED CARROT AND RICE SOUP

Ingredients

4 medium raw carrots, washed and chopped
1 onion, chopped
2 cups water
½ cup raw brown or basmati rice
1 cup water
2 tbsp. finely chopped parsley
1 tsp curry powder
½ tsp sea salt
½ tsp black pepper
1½ cups milk

Garnish: paprika

Cook carrots and onions in 2 cups water until tender. Set aside in its cooking liquid. In a second saucepan, cook rice in 1 cup of water until tender (approximately 20-25 minutes). Drain and discard the cooking liquid. Combine carrots, onions and cooking liquid in food processor or blender until smooth. Add to parsley, curry powder, pepper, cooked rice and milk. Return to saucepan and heat until just starting to boil. Remove from heat and serve, garnished with paprika.

Makes 4 servings
Each serving provides = ½ starch, 1 vegetable and ½ milk

ENJOY!

MUSHROOM AND LEEK SOUP

Ingredients

1 ½ tsp vegetable oil
1 cup chopped onion
1 leek, thinly sliced
2 ½ cups beef stock
1 cup diced peeled potatoes
1 ½ tsp margarine
12oz mushrooms, sliced
½ cup milk

In non-stick medium saucepan, heat oil; sauté garlic, onion and leek until softened, approximately 10 minutes. Add stock and potatoes; cover and simmer for 20-25 minutes or until softened. Puree in food processor until smooth. Return to saucepan and set aside.

In non-stick skillet, melt margarine; sauté mushrooms until softened, approximately 5 minutes. Add to soup and stir until combined. Stir in milk.

Makes 4 servings
Each serving provides = 1 vegetable 1 fat

ENJOY!

ORANGE BORSCHT

Ingredients

3 cups peeled and grated beets
3 cups chicken stock
1 cup unsweetened orange juice
1 cup unsweetened tomato juice
1 sprig fresh thyme or ¼ tsp dried thyme
Ground black pepper
2 tbsp. chopped parsley

Place beets and stock in saucepan and bring to a boil, simmer for 20 minutes. Strain stock into a clean saucepan and add 1 cup of the cooked beets. Discard the remaining beets. Add the juices, thyme, and pepper. Bring to a boil and remove sprig of thyme. Serve in bowls and sprinkle with parsley.

To store: cover and refrigerate for up to three days.
Makes 4 servings
Each serving provides = 1 ½ vegetable ¼ fruit

ENJOY!

PUMPKIN SOUP

Ingredients

1 ½ lb pumpkin, peeled, cut into large pieces
1 large leek, sliced
3 cups chicken stock
2 tsp mixed dried herbs or 3 tsp fresh herbs
½ tsp coarsely ground black pepper
¼ tsp ground nutmeg
¼ tsp coriander
½ tsp sea salt
2 tbsp. lemon juice
2 tbsp. chopped parsley

Place all ingredients except lemon juice and parsley in a saucepan.

Bring to a boil and simmer until pumpkin is tender (approximately 20 minutes).

Cool slightly; blend in food processor or blender until smooth.

Add lemon juice and parsley. Check taste, add sea salt if needed.

To store: cover and refrigerate for up to 3 days.

Makes 4 servings
Each serving provides = 1 vegetable

Enjoy!

BROCCOLI, BARLEY AND LEEK SOUP

Ingredients

1 tbsp. vegetable oil
2 large leeks, sliced into thin rounds
1 ½ tsp garlic, crushed
2 carrots, diced
3 ½ cups chicken stock
1/3 cup barley
2 cups chopped broccoli
½ cup milk
3 tbsp. chopped fresh dill or 1 tsp dried dill-weed

In large non-stick, saucepan, heat oil; sauté leeks, garlic and carrots until softened, 10 to 12 minutes, stirring often. Add stock, barley and broccoli; cover and simmer for 30 to 40 minutes or until barley is tender. Puree in food processor or blender until smooth and creamy. Return to pan; stir in milk and dill, blending well.

Makes 4 serving
Each serving provides = 1 veg, ½ fat, ½ starch,

Enjoy!

VEGETABLE BEEF BARLEY SOUP

Ingredients

1 tbsp. vegetable oil
2 tsp garlic, crushed
1 medium onion, diced
2 celery stalks, diced
2 carrots, diced
2 cups mushrooms, sliced
3 ½ cups beef stock
1/3 cup barley
2 small potatoes, peeled and diced
4oz stewing beef, diced
2 tbsp. chopped fresh parsley

In large non-stick saucepan, heat oil; sauté's garlic, onion, celery, carrots and mushrooms until tender, approximately 10 minutes; add stock, barley, potatoes and beef; cover, reduce heat and simmer approximately 50 minutes or until barley and potatoes are tender, stirring occasionally. Add more stock if too thick. Serve sprinkled with parsley.

Makes 4 servings
Each serving provides = 1 vegetable, ¼ protein, ¼ fat, ¼ starch

Enjoy!

ITALIAN TOMATO AND RICE SOUP

Ingredients

12oz jar chunky salsa
1 cup tomato juice
1/3 cup quick cooking brown rice
1 tbsp. dried minced onion
1 tsp Italian seasoning, crushed
1 tsp instant chicken bouillon granules
1/8 tsp dried minced garlic
1/8 tsp pepper
16oz package loose –packed frozen zucchini, carrots, cauliflower, lima beans and Italian beans.

In a large saucepan combine the salsa, tomato juice, brown rice, onion, Italian seasoning, bouillon granules, garlic, pepper and 2 cups water. Bring to a boil; reduce heat.

Cover and simmer for 10 minutes.

Meanwhile, place frozen vegetables in a colander. Run cold water over vegetables until thawed.

Stir vegetables into the rice mixture: Return to boiling, reduce heat.

Cover and simmer for 5 to 10 minutes or until rice and vegetables are tender.

Makes 6 servings = 1 cup
Each serving provides = 1 vegetable

Enjoy!

CREAMY BEAN AND CLAM CHOWDER

Ingredients

1 tbsp. vegetable oil
1 ½ cups chopped onion
2 tsp crushed garlic
5oz clams
2 cups chicken stock
1 medium potato, peeled and diced
1 ½ cups white kidney beans
2tbsp. chopped fresh dill or 5ml dried dill-weed
2 tbsp. chopped fresh chives or green onions
1 tbsp. chopped fresh parsley or (2 tsp dried)

In a non- stick saucepan, heat oil sauté's onion and garlic until softened, approximately 5 minutes

To sauce pan, add stock and potatoes; cover and simmer for 20 minutes or until potato is tender.

Add beans; cover and cook for 10 minutes.

Puree in food processor until smooth. Return to saucepan; stir in reserved clams, chives and parsley.

Makes 4 to 6 servings
Each serving provides = ½ protein, ½ vegetable, ¼ starch, 1 fat

Enjoy!

GAZPACHO

Ingredients

1 ½ cups tomato sauce
¼ cup water
1 cup chopped tomatoes
1 large clove garlic, chopped
½ tsp ground cumin
2 tbsp. red wine vinegar
1 tbsp. lemon juice
½ cup peeled, chopped cucumber
½ cup chopped green pepper
2 green onions including tops, chopped
Dash hot pepper sauce to taste (optional)
Chopped fresh parsley or chopped fresh cilantro for garnish

Directions:

Combine all ingredients except parsley or cilantro in a medium bowl.

Cover bowl, chill for several hours or overnight to allow flavors to blend.

Serve very cold, garnish with parsley or cilantro to taste sprinkled on top

Makes 4 servings
Each serving provides = 1 vegetable

Enjoy!

GOLDEN SQUASH SOUP

Ingredients

¾ cup chopped onion
½ cup chopped tomato
1 ½ cups + 2 tbsp. chicken stock
2 cups thinly sliced yellow crookneck squash (about ¾ pound)
¾ tsp crushed dried basil
¼ tsp garlic powder
¼ tsp crushed dried oregano
¼ tsp white pepper (optional)
½ cup buttermilk
1 tbsp. honey
½ tsp lemon juice

GARNISH:

4 fresh basil leaves
4 thin tomato slices
Plain yfogurt

Directions

In soup pot, combine onion and tomato, and sauté in 2 tbsp. chicken stock 5 minutes to soften vegetables.

Add remaining chicken stock, squash and spices. Bring to a boil. Cover and simmer 15 minutes or until squash is tender. Remove from heat.

Puree soup in blender with buttermilk.

Return soup to pot and stir in honey and lemon juice. Cover and set over low heat just too warm through.

Garnish each serving with a basil leaf, a thin slice of tomato and a dollop of yogurt.

Makes 4 servings
Each serving provides = 1 vegetable, 1 fat

Enjoy!

HOT BORSCHT

Ingredients

3 cups water
1 cup tomato juice
¾ cup chopped onion
1 cup shredded carrots
1 cup peeled shredded beets
1 cup shredded potatoes
2 cups shredded cabbage
1 ½ tbsp. honey
1 ½ tbsp. lemon juice
Plain yogurt for garnish

Directions:

In soup pot, combine water and tomato juice and bring to a boil.
Add vegetables, cover and simmer 30 minutes, until tender.
Remove 2 cups soup from the pot and puree in blender or food processor.
Return puree soup to pot and stir in honey and lemon juice.
Cover and simmer for 5 minutes.
Serve with yogurt for garnish

Makes 6 servings
Each serving provides = 1 vegetable, ¼ starch

Enjoy!

BROCCOLI AND LENTIL SOUP

Ingredients

1 ½ tsp vegetable oil
2 tsp crushed garlic
1 medium onion, chopped
1 celery stalk, chopped
1 large carrot, chopped
4 cups chicken stock
2 ½ cups chopped broccoli
¾ cup dried lentils
2 tbsp. cheese, grated

Directions:

In large non-stick saucepan, heat oil; sauté garlic, onion, celery and carrot until softened, approximately 5 minutes.

Add stock, broccoli and lentils; cover and simmer 30 minutes, stirring occasionally, or until lentils are tender.

Puree in food processor until creamy and smooth.

Serve sprinkled with cheese.

Makes 6 servings = ½ cup
Each serving provides = ¼ fat, 1 vegetable

Enjoy!

CHINESE SCALLOP AND SHRIMP BROTH WITH SNOW PEAS

Ingredients

4 cups chicken stock
1 ½ tsp minced fresh gingerroot
2 cups snow peas
2oz scallops, diced
2oz shrimp, diced
1 tbsp. soya sauce
1 green onion, chopped

Directions:

In medium saucepan, bring chicken stock and ginger to boil. Add snow peas, scallops, shrimp and soy sauce.

Reduce heat and simmer for 2 to 3 minutes or just until scallops are opaque and shrimp are pink.

Serve sprinkled with green onion.

Tip. Chopped broccoli or asparagus is a good substitute for snow peas.

Diced chicken can replace seafood.

Makes 4 to 6 servings
Each serving provides = ½ protein, ½ vegetable

Enjoy!

BEEF STOCK

INGREDIENTS

2 pounds beef bones
8 cups water
3 celery stalks, including leaves, chopped
2 carrots, peeled and chopped
1 large onion, quartered
2 bay leaves
4 cloves garlic, minced
6 peppercorns
2 whole cloves
½ teaspoon each ground thyme and dried marjoram
Sea salt to taste

To develop a fuller flavor and deeper color in the final stock, first place the beef bones in a roasting pan and roast at 400%F for 20 minutes.

Place roasted bones in a large pot and add all remaining ingredients.

Bring to a boil. Reduce heat to low. Cover and simmer for 4 hours.

Skim off any foam that rises to the surface.

Pour stock through a fine strainer into a bowl. Discard bones and residue.

Refrigerate stock overnight. Skim of any fat that has congealed on surface.

Pour into containers with tight fitting lids. I find ice cube holders the best freeze it and bag it in freezer bags.

Stock will keep 3-4 days if refrigerated, or several months if frozen.

Makes about 8 cups for soups and sauces

CHICKEN STOCK

Ingredients

8 cups water
1 chicken carcass or 1 chicken back (ask your butcher)
2 carrots, peeled and chopped
2 celery stalks, including leaves, chopped
1 large onion, quartered
1 leek, white part only, cleaned and sliced
5 cloves garlic, minced
½ cup chopped parsley with stems
1 bay leaf
6 peppercorns
¾ tsp ground thyme
Sea salt to taste

Combine all ingredients in a large pot. If using whole chicken carcass, crack into 2 or 3 pieces. Bring to a boil over medium-high heat. Skim off any foam that rises to surface. Reduce heat to low. Cover and simmer for 2 hours.

Pour stock into a bowl. Discard bones and residue. Refrigerate stock overnight.

Skim of any fat that has congealed on surface. Pour into containers with tight fitting lids; or ice cubes trays freeze and then bag in freezer bags.

Stock will keep 3-4 days if refrigerated, or several months if frozen

Makes about 8 cups
For soups or sauces

ENJOY!

VEGETABLE STOCK

Ingredients

8 cups water
4 celery stalks, including leaves, chopped
2 leeks, white parts only, cleaned and sliced
2 large carrots, peeled and chopped
1 large onion, quartered
1 large potato, scrubbed and chopped
1 cup chopped parsley with stems
4 cloves garlic, minced
2 bay leaves
½ tsp each, ground thyme and dried rosemary
Sea salt and pepper to taste

Combine all ingredients in a large pot. Bring to a boil over medium-high heat.

Reduce to low. Cover and let simmer for 1 hour.

Remove from heat and let cool

Cover and refrigerate overnight

The next day, pour stock through a fine strainer into a bowl. Discard residue.

Pour into containers with tight-fitting lids; or ice cube trays freeze and then freezer bag them.

Stock will keep one week in refrigerator or indefinitely if frozen

Makes about 8 cups
For soups and sauces

ENJOY!

CREAMY POTATO SALAD

Ingredients

4 medium potatoes
1 cup sliced celery
¼ cup finely chopped onions
2 tbsp. dill or sweet pickle relish
½ cup plain yogurt
2 tbsp. milk
2 tsp prepared mustard
½ tsp sea salt
¼ to ½ tsp celery seed
1 hard cooked egg, chopped
½ cup mayo

Scrub potatoes. Cook potatoes covered in boiling water for 25 to 30 minutes or until tender. Drain and cool.

Peel and cube potatoes. Transfer to a large bowl. Stir in celery, onion and pickle relish.

In a small bowl combine mayonnaise, yogurt, milk, mustard, salt and celery seed. Pour over potatoes toss to coat potatoes. Carefully fold in chopped egg.

Cover and chill for 4 to 24 hours. Serve in a lettuce lined bowl if desired.

Makes 8 servings = ½ cup
Each serving provides = 1 starch ½ fat ½ vegetable

ENJOY!

MACARONI SALAD

Ingredients

2 ½ cups cooked pasta
¾ cup plain yogurt
¼ cup chopped onion
¼ cup chopped celery
1 hard cooked egg, finely chopped
1 tbsp. prepared mustard
1 tbsp. sweet pickle relish
2 tsp sugar
½ teaspoon seasoned salt
¼ teaspoon freshly ground black pepper
Freshly chopped parsley for garnish (optional)

In large bowl, combine all ingredients until blended. Cover and refrigerate several hours or overnight. Garnish with parsley, if desired.

Makes 4 servings
Each serving = 1 cup
Each serving provides ¼ protein 1 starch ¼ vegetable

ENJOY!

VEGETABLE SALAD

Ingredients

½ cup plain yogurt
¼ cup plus 2 tbsp. mayonnaise
1 tbsp. chopped fresh parsley
4 tsp sugar (optional)
12oz cooked chick peas, rinsed and drained
1 cup sliced mushrooms
1 cup thinly sliced celery
½ cup thinly sliced carrot
½ cup chopped red onion
2 tsp plus 2 tbsp. sunflower seeds
3 cups thoroughly washed and drained spinach leaves

To prepare dressing, in a small bowl, combine yogurt, mayonnaise, parsley and sugar (if desired) until blended; set aside.

In a large bowl, combine remaining ingredients; except spinach leaves. Add reserved dressing and toss well to combine.

To serve, arrange spinach leaves on large serving platter; spoon salad mixture on top.

Makes 6 servings = ½ cup
Each serving provides = 1 fat 1 protein 2 vegetables

ENJOY!

SPINACH SALAD

Ingredients

6 cups packed fresh spinach leaves, stems removed
1 ½ cups thinly sliced mushrooms
1 cup thinly sliced red onion rings
1 can (10 ounces) mandarin oranges, drained
2 slices raw bacon
1 tbsp. lemon juice
1 clove garlic, minced
2 ½ tbsp. Honey
1 tbsp. white vinegar
1/8 tsp black pepper

Toss together spinach, mushrooms, onion rings and ½ the mandarin oranges in a large bowl. Set aside

In a small skillet, cook bacon over medium –high heat until crisp.

Shake off excess drippings and transfer bacon to a blender or food processor.

Don't discard the bacon drippings. Leave them in the skillet.

Add remaining mandarin oranges and lemon juice to bacon in blender.

Whirl briefly until oranges and bacon are pureed.

Return orange and bacon mixture to skillet with bacon drippings.

Add garlic, honey, vinegar and pepper. Mix well. Mixture should be quite warm; however, you may reheat it over medium heat, if desired.

Divide salad among 6 serving plates and drizzle warm dressing over top. Serve immediately.

Makes 6 servings
Each serving provides = 1 fat 1 vegetable ½ fruit

Enjoy!

FRUIT SALAD

Ingredients

2 cups sour cream (look for a thick brand)
T tbsp. Honey
1 tbsp. frozen orange juice concentrate
1 tsp grated orange zest
6 cups chopped fresh fruit (try a combination of bananas, oranges, kiwi fruit, strawberries and apples, (or choose your favorites.)

Mix first four ingredients together in a small bowl.
Cover and refrigerate for 1 hour
Stir sauce and fruit together in a large bowl
Serve immediately.
Makes 6 servings
Each serving provides= 1 fruit 1 fat

Hint: To prevent the flesh of apples from turning brown after cutting or peeling them, dip them in lemon juice. Make sure you mix the sauce and fruit together just before serving. Otherwise the salad will be runny

Enjoy!

CARROT AND RAISIN SALAD

Ingredients

½ cup plain yogurt
1 ½ tbsp. Honey
¼ tsp cinnamon
2 cups shredded carrots
½ cup raisins
¼ cup canned unsweetened crushed pineapple drained

In serving bowl, combine yogurt, honey, lemon juice and cinnamon into a smooth dressing. Add carrots and pineapple to dressing and stir gently, but thoroughly, until salad is uniform. Cover and chill for a minimum of 15 minutes. Toss again before serving and drain liquid, if desired. Use slotted spoon to serve.

Makes 6 servings
Each serving provides = 1 veg

Enjoy!

PICNIC MACARONI SALAD

Ingredients

3 cups cooked macaroni, cooked and drained
1/3 cup mayonnaise
1/3 cup thinly sliced celery
2 tbsp. minced fresh parsley
2 tbsp. chopped scallions
2 tbsp. chopped red bell pepper
2 hard-boiled eggs sliced
½ tsp sea salt
¼ tsp coarsely ground pepper

Mix all ingredients in a large bowl. Cover and refrigerate several hours for flavors to blend.

Makes 8 servings = ½ cup
Each serving provides = 1 starch ½ fat Enjoy!

PENNE SALAD

Ingredients

8oz penne noodles or rotini or med shell pasta for the noodles
2 ½ cups chopped tomatoes
1 cup thinly sliced sweet yellow or green pepper
½ cup chopped fresh basil or 1 ½ tsp dried
1/3 cup shredded cheese
1 tsp crushed garlic
2 tbsp. olive oil
1 tbsp. lemon juice
2 green onions sliced

Cook noodles according to package directions or until firm to the bite. Drain and place in serving bowl. Add tomatoes, yellow pepper, basil, cheese, garlic, oil, and lemon juice; toss well. Sprinkle with green onion. Chill for at least 2 hours before serving.

Makes 6 servings = ½ cup
Each serving provides = 1 starch 1 veg ¼ protein

Enjoy!

COTTAGE CHEESE AND DILL DIP

Ingredients

1 cup cottage cheese
2 tbsp. sliced green onion
2 tbsp. snipped fresh parsley
1 tsp dried dill-weed
1 tsp Worcestershire sauce
1/8 tsp pepper
Dash garlic powder

In blender container or food processor bowl place cottage cheese, Worcestershire sauce, green onion, snipped parsley, dill-weed, pepper and garlic powder. Blend until smooth. Chill covered for 1 hour before serving. Serve with an assortment of sliced raw veg or crackers.

Makes 8 servings = 2 tbsp.

Enjoy!

SPINACH VALENTINO

Ingredients

1 bunch spinach
4 mushrooms, sliced
2 shallots, sliced
2 eggs, hardboiled, sliced
1 quality orange and soy dressing

Wash spinach thoroughly, and shake gently to remove excess water. Remove the stalks and tear into bite- size pieces. Combine spinach, mushrooms, shallots and sliced eggs toss in dressing. Chill before serving

Makes 4 servings
Each serving provides = ½ protein ¾ vegetable

Enjoy!

ORANGE AND SOY DRESSING

Ingredients

¼ cup unsweetened orange juice
2 tsp soy sauce
1 clove garlic crushed
1 tsp oil (optional)
Combine all ingredients in a screw top jar
Chill and shake well before use
Cover and refrigerate for up to two days
Makes ¼ cup
2 tbsp. = 1 serving

Enjoy!

COLESLAW

Ingredients

1/3 cup plain yogurt
1 tbsp. apple cider vinegar
2 tbsp. Honey
2 cups coarsely chopped cabbage
½ cup shredded carrots
¼ cup chopped green pepper
¼ cup chopped celery

Combine yogurt, vinegar and honey in a bowl large enough to hold coleslaw. Stir until smooth and well blended. Add vegetables and mix well. Cover and chill for a minimum of 15 minutes. Toss again before serving and drain liquid, if desired. Use slotted spoon to serve.

Makes 4 serving
Each serving provides = 1 vegetable ½ fat

Enjoy!

HERBED COUSCOUS AND VEGETABLES

Ingredients

1 cup sliced fresh mushrooms
1 tbsp. margarine
1 cup water
1tbsp fresh parsley
½ tsp dried basil, crushed
¼ tsp salt
1/8 tsp dried oregano, crushed
Dash pepper
2/3 cup couscous
1 med tomato, peeled, seeded and chopped

In a medium saucepan cook mushrooms in hot margarine till tender. Carefully add water to saucepan, stir in parsley, basil, salt, oregano and pepper. Bring to a boil; remove from heat. Stir in couscous. Let stand; covered for 5 minutes. Stir in tomato

Makes 4 servings
Each serving provides = 1 starch ¼ vegetable

Enjoy!

FRUIT & PASTA SALAD

Ingredients

1 med orange
¼ cup plain yogurt
1 tsp sugar
Dash salt
¼ cup bow tie pasta cooked and drained
2 medium apple, cored and chopped
2 tbsp. sliced green onions

Finely shred orange peel to make ½ tsp set aside. Remove the remaining peel from orange and section orange over a bowl to catch juice. Measure 2 tbsp. of the juice. In a medium mixing bowl stir together orange peel, the 2 tbsp. of juice, yogurt, sugar and salt. Mix well. Add cooked pasta, chopped apples and sliced green onions; toss to coat. Gently stir in orange sections.

Cover and chill for 2 to 24 hours Makes 6 servings = ½ cup Enjoy!

COLSLAW

Ingredients

5 cups coarsely shredded green cabbage
2 cups coarsely shredded red cabbage
1 cup grated carrot
¾ cup thinly sliced celery
¼ cup each white vinegar and sugar
1 tbsp. vegetable oil
1 tsp Dijon mustard
½ tsp celery seeds
¼ tsp each sea salt and black pepper

Place first four ingredients in a very large bowl and toss until well mixed.

To prepare dressing, combine vinegar, sugar, vegetable oil, Dijon mustard, celery seeds, salt and pepper in a small saucepan.

Heat over medium –high heat until mixture comes to a boil and sugar dissolves.

Add to cabbage mixture and stir until well blended.

Cover and chill at least 2 hours before serving.

Makes 8 servings
Each serving provides 1 veg

Enjoy!

GARDEN SALAD

Ingredients

5 cups shredded / torn romaine or green leaf lettuce, or mixed greens
1 cup chopped radicchio
1 cup alfalfa sprouts
1 cup carrot grated
1 small red onion, thinly sliced into rings
8 cherry tomatoes, halved
24 thin slices unpeeled English cucumber
1 cup seasoned croutons

To assemble salad, divide lettuce among 4 serving plates. Sprinkle each with ¼ cup radicchio and ¼ cup alfalfa sprouts, followed by ¼ cup grated carrot and ¼ cup of the red onion. Arrange 4 cherry tomato halves, 6 cucumber slices and ¼ cup croutons on top.

TANGY VINAIGRETTA DRESSING

Ingredients

3 tbsp. each red wine vinegar and apple juice
2 tsp olive oil
1 clove garlic, minced
1 tsp sugar
½ tsp each Dijon mustard and dried oregano
1/8 tsp black pepper

Whisk all ingredients together in a small bowl. Serve at room temperature.

Drizzle dressing over individual salads and serve immediately.

Makes 4 servings

Enjoy!

RUSSIAN DRESSING

Ingredients

½ cup plain yogurt
2 tbsp. ketchup
1 tsp honey
2 tbsp. finely chopped green pepper
Dash hot pepper sauce
Directions

Combine all ingredients in a wide mouth jar or small bowl. Mix vigorously with a fork or wire whisk until yogurt, ketchup and honey are evenly blended.

Chill 15 minutes before serving

Store any remaining dressing in covered container in refrigerator.

Makes ¾ cup

Enjoy!

POTATO SALAD

Ingredients

10 small red potatoes, unpeeled, cut into ¼ inch thick slices (about 5 cups total)
½ cup diced carrots
¾ cup diced celery
¼ cup each diced red onions and chopped green onions
2 tbsp. chopped fresh parsley
¼ cup red wine vinegar
1 tbsp. olive oil
1 tsp sugar
½ tsp each Dijon mustard and celery seeds
1 large clove garlic, minced
¼ tsp black pepper

Steam potato slices until tender about 10 minutes. Add carrots and continue to steam for another 5-7 minutes. Drain off water.

In a large bowl, toss potatoes, carrots, celery, red onions and parsley until well mixed.

In a small bowl, whisk together vinegar, oil, sugar, Dijon mustard, celery seeds, garlic and pepper. Pour over potato mixture and stir gently until evenly coated with dressing. Serve warm or cold.

Makes 6 servings
Each serving provides = 1 starch 1 vegetable 1 fat

Enjoy!

SAVORY PASTA SALAD

Ingredients

12oz uncooked tri-color rotini (about 4 cups)
1 cup broccoli florets
½ cup carrots cut into matchsticks
½ cup each chopped sweet red and green pepper
½ cup thinly sliced mushrooms

DRESSING
Ingredients

¼ cup plus 1 tbsp. red wine vinegar
¼ cup apple juice
3 tbsp. olive oil
1 tbsp. each lemon juice and sugar
2 tsp Dijon mustard
1 large clove garlic, minced
1 tsp each dried basil and dried oregano
¼ tsp each crushed red pepper flakes, sea salt and black pepper
2 tsp parmesan cheese

Cook pasta according to package directions. Drain. Rinse well with cold water and drain again. Transfer to a large bowl.

Place broccoli and carrots in a small microwave-safe dish with ¼ cup water. Microwave on high power for 1 ½ minutes. Drain. Add to pasta along with red and green peppers and mushrooms.

Combine all dressing ingredients in a small bowl. Stir well using a whisk. Pour dressing over pasta and vegetables. Stir well to coat pasta with dressing. Cover and refrigerate for 4 hours before serving.

Tastes even better the next day!

Makes 8 servings
Each serving provides = 1 starch 1 vegetable 1 fat

Enjoy!

RICE SALAD

Ingredients

1 cup uncooked long grain rice. Make sure the brown rice you're using is the quicker cooking variety (cooks in 25 minutes), but not minute rice
1 cup orange juice
1-1/3 cups chicken stock
1 ½ cups diced cantaloupe
1 cup peeled and diced English cucumber
½ cup each diced sweet red pepper and chopped green onions
2 tbsp. chopped fresh coriander

DRESSING
Ingredients

3 tbsp. lime juice
2 tbsp. Honey
1 tbsp. olive oil
1 tsp prepared mustard
1 clove garlic, minced
½ tsp. ground cumin
3-4 dashes hot pepper sauce
¼ tsp sea salt

Combine rice, orange juice and chicken stock in a medium saucepan. Bring to a boil. Reduce heat to medium –low. Cover and simmer until rice is tender and all the liquid has been absorbed, about 25 minutes. Let rice cool completely.

In a large bowl, stir together rice, cantaloupe, cucumber, red pepper, green onions and coriander. In a small bowl, whisk together all dressing ingredients. Pour over rice mixture and stir well

Cover and refrigerate for 1 hour before serving.

Makes 8 servings
Each serving provides= 1 starch 1 vegetable 1 fat ½ fruit

Enjoy!

CALIFORNIA – STYLE SALAD

Ingredients

6oz uncooked rotini or other shaped pasta (about 2 cups dry)
2 cups chopped cooked chicken breast
1 cup diced celery
1 cup mandarin orange sections (try apples if you don't like mandarins)
½ cup water chestnuts cut into slivers
2 tbsp. chopped fresh parsley
¾ cup plain yogurt
2 tbsp. honey
1 tbsp. frozen orange juice concentrate
1 tsp poppy seeds
½ tsp dry; mustard
¼ tsp black pepper
Lettuce (any kind you like)

Cook pasta according to package directions. Drain and rinse with cold water.

Transfer pasta to a large bowl. Add chicken, celery, orange sections, water chestnuts and parsley. Mix well.

In separate bowl, stir together yogurt, honey, orange juice concentrate, poppy seeds, mustard and pepper. Pour yogurt mixture over chicken/pasta mixture and toss. Serve on a bed of lettuce.

Makes 4 servings
Each serving provides = 1 protein 1 starch 1 vegetable 1 fat ½ fruit

Enjoy!

If you don't have any chicken on hand, try tuna, turkey, crabmeat or shrimp in its place.

CHICKEN SALAD

Ingredients

2 cups chopped cooked chicken breast
1 cup canned black beans, drained and rinsed
1 ½ cups diced tomato
1 cup whole kernel corn
½ cup diced red onions
¼ cup chopped fresh coriander

DRESSING
Ingredients

2 tbsp. lime juice
1 tbsp. olive oil
½ tsp each; ground cumin and sugar
¼ tsp each; sea salt and black pepper

Combine first 6 ingredients in a large bowl and mix well
In a small bowl, whisk together dressing ingredients
Pour over bean mixture until dressing is evenly distributed
Cover and refrigerate until ready to serve

Makes 6 servings
Each serving provides = 1 protein 1 vegetable ¼ fat

Enjoy!

TABBOULEH GREEK SALAD

Ingredients

¾ cup Bulgur
½ cup finely chopped onion
1 cup diced cucumber
1 ½ cups diced tomato
2 green onions, sliced thinly
¼ cup sliced pitted black olives
2oz feta cheese crumbled

DRESSING
Ingredients

1/3 cup chopped fresh parsley
1/3 cup chopped fresh mint
2 tbsp. lemon juice
2 tbsp. vegetable oil
1 tsp crushed garlic
¾ tsp dried basil
½ tsp dried oregano

Cover bulgur with 2 cups boiling water; soak for 20 minutes, drain well and place in a large serving bowl. Add onion, cucumber, tomatoes, green onions, olives and feta cheese; mix well.

Dressing: in a small bowl, combine parsley, mint, lemon juice, oil, garlic, basil and oregano; pour over Tabbouleh. Mix well, refrigerate until chilled.

Makes 4-6 servings
Each serving provides = 1 vegetable 1 starch

Enjoy!

WARM CHICKEN SALAD WITH ORANGE DRESSING

TUM YUM!

Ingredients

1 ½ cups snow peas, sliced in half
8oz boneless skinless chicken breast, cubed
1 large head romaine lettuce, torn
1 cup mandarin orange segments
½ cup sliced water chestnuts
2 tbsp. pecans

DRESSING
Ingredients

2 tsp grated orange rind
¼ cup orange juice
½ tsp crushed garlic
1 tbsp. frozen orange juice concentrate, thawed
2 tbsp. mayonnaise
3 tbsp. vegetable oil
1tbsp. chopped tarragon (or 1 tsp dried)

Dressing: In a small bowl, whisk together orange rind and juice, garlic, orange juice concentrate, mayonnaise, oil and tarragon until well blended. Set aside.

Steam or microwave snow peas just until tender- crisp. Drain and place in salad bowl. In saucepan, pour in just enough water to cover chicken; bring to a boil. Reduce heat, cover and simmer for 2 to 3 minutes or until chicken is no longer pink; drain and add to snow peas. Add lettuce, oranges, and chestnuts to salad bowl. Pour dressing over top and toss. Sprinkle with pecans

Makes 6 servings
Each serving provides = ½ protein 1 vegetable 1 fat ½ fruit

Enjoy!

CREAMY CUCUMBER SALAD

Ingredients

1 large cucumber, peeled
1 cup plain yogurt
2 tsp white or cider vinegar
1 tbsp. snipped fresh dill or 1 tsp dried dill weed
½ tsp sea salt
¼ tsp freshly ground pepper

Slice cucumber lengthwise and remove seeds. Thinly slice cucumber and place in a salad bowl. Add remaining ingredients. Mix thoroughly and chill at least ½ hour before serving.

Makes 5 servings = each serving = ½ cup
Each serving provides = 1 veg

Enjoy!

CUCUMBER DILL SAUCE

Ingredients

½ cup plain yogurt
¼ small cucumber, seeded and diced
½ small tomato, diced fine
1 tbsp. finely chopped onion
1 tbsp. fresh dill or ¾ tsp dried dill

To prepare sauce, combine yogurt, cucumber, tomato, onion and dill in a small bowl mix well

Enjoy!

COTTAGE CHEESE AND DILL DIP

Ingredients

1 cup cottage cheese 2%
2 tbsp. sliced green onion
2 tbsp. snipped fresh parsley
1 tsp dried dill weed
1 tsp Worcestershire sauce
1/8 tsp pepper
Dash garlic powder

In blender container or food processor bowl place cottage cheese, Worcestershire sauce, green onion, snipped parsley, dill weed, pepper and garlic powder. Blend until smooth; chill, covered for 1 hour before serving.

Serve with an assortment of sliced raw vegetables or crackers.

Makes 8 servings = 2 tbsp.

Enjoy!

COTTAGE CHEESE AND APPLE SNACKS

Ingredients

1 cup cottage cheese 2%
2 tbsp. peanut butter
¼ tsp ground cinnamon or apple pie spice
1 to 2 tsp milk
3 medium apples or pears, cored and sliced

FOR DIP- In a blender or food processor bowl place cottage cheese, peanut butter, cinnamon or apple pie spice. Cover and blend or process till smooth. If necessary, stir in enough milk to make dip of desired consistency.

Serve the dip immediately or cover and chill it for up to 24 hours.

Serve dip with the apple or pear slices.

To keep apple or pear slices from turning brown brush them with a little lemon juice.

Makes 6 servings = 2 tbsp.

Enjoy!

FRUITY COTTAGE CHEESE SALAD

Ingredients

½ cup cottage cheese 2%
1 small apple chopped = ½ cup
2 tbsp. mixed dried fruit bits or raisins
2 tsp mayonnaise or salad dressing
Dash, ground cinnamon, ground nutmeg or apple pie spice
1 lettuce leaf

In an airtight container stir together cottage cheese, apple dried fruit bits, mayonnaise and cinnamon. Chill overnight.

Pack 1 lettuce leaf in a small clear plastic bag. Carry with the container of cottage cheese mixture in an insulated lunch box with a frozen ice pack.

Serve cottage cheese mixture atop lettuce leaf.

Makes 12 serving
Each serving provides = 1 protein 1 fruit 1 fat

Enjoy!

SOUTH WEST DRESSING

Ingredients

½ cup plain yogurt
2 tbsp. ketchup
1 tsp honey
½ tsp chilli powder
Dash hot pepper sauce
2 tbsp. chopped fresh cilantro (optional)
¼ cup chopped tomato

Combine all ingredients in blender or food processor: Process for a few seconds at a time; using pulsing motion; in order to blend all ingredients, yet retain some tomato texture.

Chill 15 minutes before serving. Store any remaining dressing in covered container in refrigerator.

Makes ¾ cup

Enjoy!

GINGER PEARS

Ingredients

4 medium pears, peeled and quartered
10oz ginger ale
Juice of 1 lemon
½ tsp minced fresh ginger
¼ cup orange juice (concentrate)
3-4 drops yellow food coloring (optional)
5 cloves
Ground cinnamon

Directions:

Place pears in saucepan. Add ginger ale, lemon juice, ginger, orange juice concentrate, food coloring, and cloves.

Cover and simmer until pears are tender, turning and basting the pears to they cook evenly. Alternatively microwave: covered, on high for 4-6 minutes until tender lift pears onto serving dish. Simmer juices until slightly reduced

Pour over pears. Sprinkle with cinnamon. Serve hot or chilled.

To store: cover and refrigerate for up to four days.

Makes 4 servings
Each serving provides = 1 ¼ fruits

Enjoy!

ORANGE SAUCE

Ingredients

1 ½ tsp margarine
1 ½ tsp all-purpose flour
¾ cup orange juice
½ tsp grated orange rind

In small saucepan, melt margarine; stir in flour and cook, stirring for 1 minute. Add orange juice and rind; cook stirring, until thickened.

Makes ¾ cup; 1 tbsp. per serving
Use over cooked chicken, turkey or Cornish hens.

Enjoy!

GINGER LEMON MARINADE

Ingredients

3 tbsp. lemon juice
2 tbsp. water
1 tbsp. vegetable oil
1 ½ tsp red wine vinegar
4 tsp brown sugar
2 tsp sesame oil
1 tsp minced gingerroot (or ¼ tsp ground ginger)
½ tsp ground coriander
½ tsp ground fennel seeds (optional)

Directions:

In small bowl, combine lemon juice, water, vegetable oil, vinegar, sugar, sesame oil, ginger, coriander and fennel seeds (if using); mix well.

Makes ½ cup = 1 tbsp. per serving

Use to marinate chicken, fish or veal. Remove meat and broil for 3 to 5 minutes until thickened. Brush over meat before cooking.

Enjoy!

CHERRY SAUCE

Ingredients

2 cups fresh ripe cherries, pitted
½ cup chicken stock
1 tsp Worcestershire sauce
1 tbsp. brandy

Directions: place 1 cup of cherries into a saucepan or in a microwave bowl with stock and Worcestershire sauce. Boil for 8 minutes until cherries are soft, or microwave on high for 4 minutes. Puree and return to saucepan or bowl. Add remaining cup of cherries and brandy. Simmer for 2 minutes or microwave on high for 2 minutes, and serve.

Makes 2 cups
Each serving provides = ½ fruit

Enjoy!

RATATOUILLE SAUCE

Ingredients

1 small green bell pepper, diced
1 small eggplant peeled, and diced
2 small zucchini, diced
2 medium tomatoes, diced, or 16 cherry tomatoes
6 medium mushrooms, diced
1 large onion, peeled, and diced
1 clove garlic, crushed
½ tsp dried oregano
Black pepper to taste
3 tbsp. water

Directions:

Combine all ingredients and cook over low heat for 30 minutes, or microwave on medium for 15 minutes.

Makes 4 servings
Each serving provides = 2 vegetables

Ratatouille can be served as a hot vegetable or chilled as a salad. It is also ideal to surround chicken, veal or fish fillets during cooking.

Enjoy!

THICK AND RICH TOMATO SAUCE

Ingredients

1 tbsp. vegetable oil
2 tsp crushed garlic
½ cup chopped onion
½ cup chopped sweet green onion
½ cup chopped carrots
1 can (28oz) canned crushed tomatoes
¼ cup red wine
2 tbsp. tomato paste
1 bay leaf
1 tsp dried oregano
1 tsp dried basil

Directions: In large non-stick saucepan, heat oil; sauté onion, green pepper and carrots until softened, approximately 10 minutes. Add tomatoes, wine, tomato paste, bay leaf, oregano and basil; cover and simmer for approximately 30 minute, stirring occasionally.

Discard bay leaf. Puree if desired.

Make the day before or freeze for up to 6 weeks.

Makes 3 cups = 1/3 cup
Each serving provides 1 vegetable, ¼ fat

Enjoy!

SIZZLIN' SALSA

Ingredients

6 cups seeded and diced tomatoes (fresh not canned)
2 cups diced onions
6 cloves garlic, minced
5 jalapeno peppers (seeded and minced)
1 cup tomato sauce
1 tbsp. ground cumin
½ tsp each paprika and sea salt
2 tbsp. red wine vinegar or cider vinegar
1/8 tsp cayenne pepper (or to taste)
½ cup chopped fresh coriander
3 tbsp. lime juice (preferable fresh)

Combine tomatoes, onions, garlic, and jalapenos in a large saucepan.
Cook over medium-high heat for about 10 minutes, stirring often.
Stir in tomato sauce, cumin, paprika, vinegar, salt and cayenne pepper.
Continue to cook for another 10 minutes.
Remove from heat. Add coriander and lime juice. Mix well.
Serve when cool.

Makes 8 cups
Each serving provides = 1 vegetable

Enjoy!

RUSSIAN DRESSING

Ingredients

½ cup plain yogurt
2 tbsp. ketchup
1 tsp honey
2 tbsp. finely chopped green pepper
Dash hot pepper sauce

Combine all ingredients in a wide mouth jar or small bowl. Mix vigorously with a fork or wire whisk until yogurt, ketchup and honey are evenly blended. Chill 15 minutes before serving. Store any remaining dressing in covered container in refrigerator.

Makes ¾ cup Enjoy!

HUMMAS

Ingredients

¼ cup water
1 cup drained canned chick peas
¾ tsp crushed garlic
2 tbsp. lemon juice
4 tsp olive oil
¼ cup tahini
1 tbsp. chopped fresh parsley

In food processor, combine water, chick peas, garlic, lemon juice, oil and tahini.

Process until creamy and smooth.

Transfer to serving dish; sprinkle with parsley.

Makes 1 cup serves 4 to 6
Each serving provides ¼ protein and ½ fat

Enjoy!

MUSHROOM SAUCE

Ingredients

1 tbsp. margarine
1 ½ cups sliced mushrooms
2 tbsp. all-purpose flour
½ cup chicken or beef stock
½ cup milk
1 tbsp. sherry (optional)

In small non-stick saucepan, melt margarine; sauté mushrooms until tender, approximately 3 minutes. Add flour and stir until combined.

Add stock and milk; cook on low heat, stirring constantly, until thickened, 4 to 5 minutes. Add sherry (if using). If too thick add more milk.

Makes 1 ½ cups =¼ cup = 1 serving
Each serving provides = vegetable ½ fat

Enjoy!

SALSA

Ingredients

2 medium tomatoes
½ medium onion
½ medium green pepper
1 small fresh jalapeno pepper (optional)
¼ cup fresh cilantro leaves
1 tbsp. line or lemon juice
1 tbsp. apple cider vinegar
1 clove garlic, split
¼ tsp chilli powder
¼ tsp cumin

DIRECTIONS:

Cut vegetables into pieces of about equal size ½ inch or smaller

Combine all ingredients, put aside ½ cup mixture. Put remaining mixture in blender or food processor. Using pulsing: (on-off) motion process to desired texture: The optimum salsa has an uneven coarse consistency, rather than a paste or puree. If you do not have a food processor and wish to do this by hand, chop vegetables as fine as possible and combine with remaining ingredients.

Add ½ cup mixture back into blended salsa and stir. This will provide chunkier texture.

Transfer to shallow serving dish. Chill for 15 minutes before serving.

To keep for more than a day or two, bring salsa to a boil, then transfer to covered container and chill.

Salsa should be used within a week.
Makes 1 ¼ cups

Enjoy!

CHIP-CHIP HOORAY

Ingredients

1 tbsp. olive oil or vegetable oil
1 egg white
4 6-inch whole wheat pitas
Mixed herb seasoning
Preheat oven to 350%F

Whisk together olive oil and egg white in a small bowl. Set aside

Using scissors cut the pitas in half. Open up the pockets, and cut each half into 2 half circles. Stack half circles 2 at a time; then cut into 3 wedges. You should end up with 12 chips from each whole pita.

Using a pastry brush, lightly brush the inside of each pita chip with olive oil mixture.

Place chips on a baking sheet, oil side up, in a single layer. Sprinkle herb seasoning over each chip.

Bake for 15 minutes, or until golden brown and crispy. (If you bite into the chip and it's chewy, that means they're not done yet.

Store chips in an airtight container or plastic bag.

Makes 4 servings
Each serving provides = 1 starch 1 fat

Enjoy!

If you love chips, but not the fat: This slimmed-down version is where it's at.

Great for snacking dunking too:
These guiltless chips are good for you!

PITA PIZZA

Ingredients

4 small whole wheat pita rounds
1 cup tomato & basil sauce or 1 cup commercial pasta sauce
3 large tomatoes, sliced
1 medium green pepper, seeded & sliced
1 cup mushrooms, sliced
1 medium onion, peeled and sliced
8 tbsp. grated cheddar cheese

HEAT OVEN TO 350%F PREP TIME 30 MINUTES

Spread each pita round with sauce; arrange the vegetables evenly over the top and sprinkle with grated cheese.

Place on a lightly oiled baking tray. Bake for 20 minutes: or until cheese melts and begins to brown.

Serve pita pizzas straight from the oven, accompanied by a toss salad.

To store: prepare pizzas in advance uncooked; wrap in plastic wrap or slide into big freezer bags and freeze until needed; then place the frozen pizzas on a baking tray and bake for 25 minutes.

Makes 4 servings
Each serving provides = 1 protein 1 starch 1 vegetable

Enjoy!

VEGETABLE CURRY

Ingredients

1 lb mixed vegetables
2 tsp olive oil
1 onion sliced
1 tsp ground turmeric
½ tsp ground cumin
¾ inch; piece green ginger, chopped
1 or 2 fresh hot chilies or chili powder to taste
1 cup water
1 cup coconut milk
1 tbsp. lemon juice

Trim vegetables and cut into pieces
Heat oil until very hot in wok or large frying pan
Add onion and spices and toss until onion is golden brown
Add the rest of vegetables and stir fry for 2-3 minutes
Add 1 cup of water and cook 6-8 minutes, uncovered, or until vegetables are tender.
Add coconut milk and bring to a boil.
Remove from heat. Add lemon juice

Serve with brown rice.

Makes 4 servings
Each serving provides = 1 ½ vegetables 1 fat

Enjoy!

BULGUR PALAF

Ingredients

1 can 14 ½oz tomatoes: cut up
¼ cup sliced green onions
1 tsp chicken stock
½ tsp dried thyme, crushed
1 cup Bulgur
¼ cup raisins

Drain tomatoes, reserving juice. Add enough water to juice to equal 2 cups. Set aside.

In a medium saucepan combine tomato, juice-water mixture, green onions, chicken stock and thyme.

Bring mixture to boiling; add bulgur. Cover and simmer for 12 minutes. Stir in tomatoes and raisins. Cover and simmer for 3 to 5 minutes more or till bulgur is tender and all the liquid is absorbed.

Makes 6 servings = ½ cup
Each serving provides = 1 starch

Enjoy!

HONEY MUSTARD MIXED VEGETABLES

Ingredients

½ cup carrots; cut in thin 2-inch sticks
1 ½ cups broccoli and cauliflower
2 tbsp. Dijon mustard
2 tbsp. honey
½ tsp dried dill weed

Steam carrots for 10 minutes: add cauliflower & broccoli and steam until tender, approximately 8 additional minutes

Combine mustard with honey and dill to make a smooth sauce

Mix sauce with hot cooked vegetables and stir gently until sauce is evenly distributed.

Makes 4 servings
Each serving provides 1 vegetable ½ fat Enjoy!

FRESH STRAWBERRY CONSERVE

Ingredients

½ pint strawberries, hulled and roughly chopped
1 level tsp gelatin soaked in 1 ½ tbsp. Water
1 tbsp. lemon juice
4 level tsp sugar

Place strawberries in saucepan with water and lemon juice. Cover and bring to a boil and simmer for 10 minutes. Mash fruit slightly and let stand for 10 minutes.

Dissolve gelatin according to instructions on packet, and add to fruit. Stir in sugar. Pour into a clean hot jar. Cover and refrigerate: Up to two weeks.

You can vary this recipe by using other berries instead of strawberries

1 tbsp. = 1 serving

Free food

Enjoy!

SLIM DUNK

Ingredients

2 cups sour cream
¼ cup mayonnaise
1 -10oz package frozen spinach, thawed, squeezed dry, and chopped
1 envelope 77 grams "Knorr" brand leek soup mix
¼ cup minced sweet red pepper
Combine all ingredients in a medium bowl. Stir well.
Cover and refrigerate for 3 hours before serving.

Makes about 3 cups

This dip tastes great served with your favorite fresh vegetables for dunking. You could also spoon the dip into a hollowed out pumpernickel loaf, chop the scooped out bread into large chunks, and use these for dunking.

Serious yum factor!

Enjoy!

BUTTERMILK YOGURT DRESSING

Ingredients

¼ cup buttermilk
¼ cup plain yogurt
2 tbsp. apple cider vinegar
1 tbsp. lemon juice
2 tsp honey
1 tsp chopped garlic
2 tbsp. chopped green onion
Pinch white pepper (optional)
½ tsp celery seed

Combine all ingredients in wide mouth jar or small bowl. Mix well until uniformly blended. Chill for 15 minutes before serving. Store any remaining dressing in covered container in refrigerator.

Makes 2/3 cup

Enjoy!

MUSTARD – DILL SAUCE

Ingredients

¾ cup plain yogurt
¼ cup prepared mustard, spicy or Dijon
1 tsp dried dill weed
½ tsp onion powder
½ tsp honey

Mix ingredients thoroughly in a small bowl. Serve on vegetables or fish.

Store any remaining sauce in covered container in refrigerator'

Makes 1 cup

Enjoy!

CREAMY ORANGE DRESSING

Ingredients

¼ cup unsweetened orange juice
2 tsp orange zest
1 tbsp. finely chopped parsley
2 tsp finely chopped chives
½ cup plain yogurt

Combine all ingredients and chill
To store: cover and refrigerate for up to two days
Makes ¾ cup: Each serving = 2 tbsp.

Enjoy!

CURRY DRESSING

Ingredients

½ cup plain yogurt
2 tsp hot curry powder
2 tbsp. chopped parsley
¼ tsp minced garlic

Mix all ingredients and adjust flavorings to taste: Chill and use the same day.

Makes ½ cup: = each serving =2 tbsp.

Enjoy!

ORANGE AND SOY DRESSING

¼ cup unsweetened orange juice
2 tsp low-sodium soy sauce
1 clove garlic, crushed

Combine all ingredients in a screw top jar. Chill and shake well before use.

To store: cover and refrigerate for up to two days.

Makes ¼ cup = each serving = 2 tbsp.

Enjoy!

CREAMY YOGURT DRESSING

Ingredients

1/3 cup plain yogurt
2 tbsp. lemon juice or raspberry vinegar
½ tsp dry mustard
Ground black pepper

Mix all ingredients until smooth. Cover and refrigerate for up to three days.

Makes ½ cup
Each serving = 2 tbsp.

Enjoy!

SWEET AND SPICY POP CORN

Ingredients

Non-stick spray coating
6 cups popped popcorn using no oil
2 tbsp. sugar
2 tsp water
¼ tsp ground cinnamon
1/8 tsp ground nutmeg
1/8 tsp ground ginger

Spray a cold 13+9+2 inch baking pan with non-stick coating. Place popcorn in the baking pan. In a small bowl stir together sugar, water, cinnamon, nutmeg and ginger. Add spice mixture to popcorn in baking pan. Toss popcorn till coated. Bake in a 350%F oven for 15 minutes, stirring once or twice. Transfer popcorn from baking pan to a large piece of foil. Cool completely. If desired, store in a tightly covered container.

Makes 6 servings = ¾ cup

Enjoy!

CURRY PASTE

Ingredients

1 tbsp. freshly minced or grated ginger
2 tbsp. ground coriander
1 tbsp. ground cinnamon
2 tsp chilli powder
1 tbsp. powdered turmeric
1 tsp minced garlic
1 tbsp. lemon juice
2 tbsp. vinegar
2 tbsp. olive oil
1 tbsp. dry mustard

Combine all ingredients in saucepan and mix to make a smooth paste. Stirring constantly, cook over low heat for 3-4 minutes until slightly thickened.

Spoon mixture; into a warm glass jar.

To store: keep in airtight container in refrigerator for up to one month.
Makes ¾ cup

CURRY POWDER

Ingredients ½ tsp cayenne pepper

2 tbsp. ground coriander
1 tbsp. ground cumin
1 tbsp. coarsely ground black pepper
2 tbsp. ground ginger
1 tbsp. ground cinnamon
½ tsp ground cloves
¼ tsp ground nutmeg
2 tsp chili powder
2 tbsp. powdered turmeric

You can vary the ingredients and quantities, according to taste.

Curry powder can be stored for a long time, but gradually loses its flavor.

Mix ingredients well. Refrigerate in airtight container.

Makes ¾ cup

Enjoy!

FRESH MANGO CHUTNEY

Ingredients

1 ripe medium- large mango
2 tsp lemon juice
½ tsp finely chopped or minced fresh ginger
1 tbsp. raisins

Peel mango, slice flesh from stone and cut into small pieces. Place in a mixing bowl. Add lemon juice, ginger and raisins.

Spoon into glass or plastic container, cover and refrigerate.

To store: keep in glass or plastic container and refrigerate for up to two days.

Makes 1 cup

PLUM SAUCE

Ingredients

2 onions, chopped
1 cup water
2lb fresh plums, pitted
1 cup fresh orange juice
2 tsp grated or minced fresh ginger
6 whole cloves
1 tsp peppercorns
Pinch of thyme
Pinch of oregano
1 bay leaf

Lightly sauté onions in 2-3 tablespoons of water for 2 minutes; Add the rest of the ingredients and cook over low heat, stirring regularly. Simmer, with the lid off for at least 1 hour until the mixture thickens. Remove the bay leaf.

Pour into clean warmed jars, cool and then seal the jars.

To store: keep sealed jars in refrigerator.

Makes 8 cups = serving =1cup

Each serving provides ¼ vegetable 1 fruit

Enjoy!

TOMATO RELISH

Ingredients

3 large onions, chopped
5 ½ lbs chopped, ripe tomatoes
5 granny smith apples, cored and chopped (skins left on)
3 cups vinegar
1 lb raisins
3 cloves of garlic, crushed
1 cup fresh orange juice
1 tsp mixed spice
1 tsp whole cloves
1 tsp chili powder

Place all ingredients in a large saucepan and bring them to a boil. Turn the heat to low and simmer for 1 hour, stirring frequently, remove from heat.

Pour hot water into clean jars to warm them. Pour water away.

Fill jars with hot relish. Allow them to cool, then seal the jars and store.

To store: keep in sealed jars. Once opened; store in refrigerator.

Makes 8 cups
1 cup provides 1 ¾ vegetable 2 fruits

Enjoy!

SOUTH WEST DRESSING

Ingredients

½ cup plain yogurt
2 tbsp. ketchup
1 tsp honey
½ tsp chili powder
Dash hot pepper sauce
2 tbsp. chopped fresh cilantro (optional)
¼ cup chopped tomato

Combine all ingredients in blender or food processor. Process for a few seconds at a time; using a pulsing motion in order to blend all ingredients; yet retain some tomato texture. Chill 15 minutes before serving. Store any remaining dressing in covered container in refrigerator.

Makes ¾ cup

Enjoy!

BUTTERMILK YOGURT DRESSING

Ingredients

¼ cup buttermilk
¼ cup plain yogurt
2 tbsp. apple cider vinegar
1 tbsp. lemon juice
2 tsp honey
1 tsp chopped garlic
2 tbsp. chopped green onion
Pinch white pepper (optional)
½ tsp celery seed

Combine all ingredients in wide mouth jar or small bowl. Mix well until uniformly blended. Chill 15 minutes before serving.

Store any remaining dressing in covered container in refrigerator.

Makes 2/3 cup

MUSTARD- DILL SAUCE

Ingredients

¾ cup plain yogurt
¼ cup prepared mustard, spicy or Dijon
1 tsp dried dill weed
½ tsp onion powder
½ tsp honey

Mix ingredients thoroughly in a small bowl. Serve on vegetables or fish.

Store any remaining sauce in covered container in refrigerator.

Makes 1 cup

CREAMY YOGURT DRESSING

Ingredients

1/3 cup plain yogurt
2 tbsp. lemon juice or raspberry vinegar
½ tsp dry mustard
Ground black pepper to taste

Mix all ingredients until smooth, cover and refrigerate. To store: cover and refrigerate for up to three days.

Makes ½ cup
Each serving = 2 tbsp.

ITALIAN DRESSING

Ingredients

1/3 cup vinegar
1 tbsp. lemon juice
1 tbsp. chopped parsley
2 tsp chopped chives
1 clove garlic, crushed
½ tsp dry mustard
Ground black pepper to taste

Combine ingredients in a screw top jar, shake well and refrigerate. To store: cover and refrigerate for up to one week.

Makes ½ cup

HERBED TOMATO DRESSING

Ingredients

½ cup unsweetened tomato juice
4 tbsp. tomato paste
2 tbsp. plain yogurt
4 drops tabasco sauce
1 clove garlic, crushed
1 tbsp. chopped parsley
½ tsp chopped fresh herbs or ¼ tsp mixed dried herbs

Use herbs such as marjoram, basil or thyme

Combine tomato juice with tomato paste and add to yogurt. Add other ingredients and mix well. Chill and use same day.

Makes 1 cup each serving = 2 tbsp. = ½ vegetable

FRESH MANGO CHUTNEY

Ingredients

1 ripe large mango
2 tsp lemon juice
½ tsp finely chopped or minced fresh ginger
1 tbsp. raisins

Peel mango. Slice flesh from stone and cut into small pieces. Place in a mixing bowl. Add lemon juice, ginger and raisins. Spoon into glass or plastic container, cover and refrigerate.

To store: keep in glass or plastic container and refrigerate for up to two days.

Makes 1 cup - each cup provides 1 ½ fruit

CRANBERRY PUNCH

Ingredients

2- 24oz bottles unsweetened white grape juice
2-12oz cans frozen cranberry juice cocktail concentrate, thawed
3-16oz bottles lemon-lime carbonated beverage
Ice ring

In a large punch bowl combine white grape juice and cranberry juice cocktail concentrate. Just before serving stir in lemon-lime carbonated beverage. Add ice ring.

Makes 30 (4oz) servings

Ice ring

Fill a 6-cup ring mold half full of water; freeze till firm about 4 hours. Cut 3 orange slices in half; arrange atop frozen ice layer. Garnish with whole cranberries and lemon leaves. Add enough water to just cover the oranges, cranberries and lemon leaves. Freeze till firm about 2 hours.

Enjoy!

SPANISH RICE

Ingredients

1 cup water
¾ cup chopped green pepper
½ cup chopped onion
½ cup chopped celery
½ tsp sea salt
1-14oz Can tomatoes cut up
¾ cup long grain rice
1 tsp chili powder
1/8 tsp pepper
Dash bottled hot pepper sauce

In medium saucepan combine water, green pepper, onion, celery and salt.

Bring to a boil, reduce heat, cover and simmer for 5 minutes.

Stir in un-drained tomatoes, rice, chili powder, pepper and hot pepper sauce.

Return to boiling; reduce heat. Cover and simmer for about 20 minutes or until rice is tender and liquid is absorbed.

Makes 6 servings = ½ cup
Each serving provides 1 starch 1 vegetable

Enjoy!

BULGAR PILAF

Ingredients

1 Can 14 ½oz can tomatoes, cut up
¼ cup sliced green onions
1 tsp instant chicken bouillon granules
½ tsp dried thyme, crushed
1 cup bulgur
¼ cup raisins

Drain tomatoes, reserving juice. Add enough water to juice to equal 2 cups. Set aside. In medium saucepan combine tomato, juice water mixture, green onions, bouillon, granules and thyme. Bring mixture to a boil; add bulgur. Cover and simmer for 12 minutes. Stir in tomatoes and raisins. Cover and simmer for 3 to 5 minutes more or till bulgur is tender and all the liquid is absorbed.

Makes 6 servings = ½ cup

Each serving provides = 1 starch Enjoy!

CHICKEN QUESADILLAS

Ingredients

1 cup canned chickpeas, drained, rinsed and mashed
½ cup sour cream
½ cup salsa (mild, hot or medium)
1 large clove garlic, minced
8- 7 inch flour tortillas
2 tsp vegetable oil
1 chicken breast, cooked and shredded
¼ cup each finely chopped sweet red pepper and chopped green onions
1 tbsp. chopped fresh coriander
1 cup shredded Monterey jack cheese (4 ounces)

Preheat oven to 400%F

Combine mashed chickpeas, 2 tbsp. sour cream, 2 tbsp. salsa and garlic in a small bowl. Mix well. Set aside.

Brush on side of each tortilla with oil. Arrange 4 tortillas, oil side down, on a baking sheet. Spread ¼ chickpea mixture over each tortilla, leaving ½ inch border.

Combine shredded chicken, red pepper, green onions and coriander in a small bowl. Spread ¼ chicken mixtures over chickpeas, followed by cheese.

Cover with remaining tortillas, oil side up.

Bake for 8 to 10 minutes, until tortillas are a light golden brown.

Remove from oven. Let cool 5 minutes before cutting (this is important) otherwise tortillas will slide apart.

Cut each quesadilla into 6 wedges.

Serve with remaining sour cream

Makes 24 wedges = 3 per serving
Each serving provides = 1 protein, 1 starch, 1 fat, 1 vegetable

Enjoy!

SWEET AND SOUR CHBBAGE & BEANS

Ingredients

¾ pound cabbage cut into strips ½ inch wide = 6 cups
1 cup no salt tomato juice
1 tbsp. lemon juice
1 tbsp. apple cider vinegar
1 tbsp. apple juice concentrates
2 tbsp. honey
1 tsp Dijon mustard
¼ cup raisins
1 large clove garlic, chopped
¼ tsp celery seed
1 tsp onion powder
Dash white pepper (optional)
1 ½ cups cooked great northern beans, drained

Directions

In large saucepan, combine all ingredients, except beans.
Bring cabbage mixture to a boil while stirring. Cover and simmer 10 minutes.
Add beans to cabbage and cook 5 minutes to heat through.

Makes 4 servings
Each serving provides = 1 protein 1 vegetable 1 fat

Enjoy!

BUBBLE AND SQUEAK

Ingredients

1 medium onion, finely sliced
2 tsp oil
4 cups cooked, mixed vegetables (e.g. potato, cabbage, pumpkin, carrot, cauliflower, broccoli, beans, peas, spinach and zucchini). Black pepper; to taste.

In frying pan, heat oil. Add onion and sauté gently until lightly browned. Add mixed vegetables and pepper. Use a metal spatula to lift and turn mixture until well combined. Then press down vegetables to make a flat cake in the frying pan. Cook over medium heat for 5 minutes, or until the bottom of the cake is well browned. Cut into wedges in the frying pan. Serve brown side up.

Makes 4 servings
Each serving provides = ½ fat & 2 vegetables Enjoy!

MICROWAVE MAIN DISH
STEAMED SOLE IN CABBAGE

Ingredients

1 pound fresh sole or other fish fillets
3 medium cabbage leaves or savoy cabbage
¾ cup shredded cabbage
½ cup shredded zucchini
1/3 cup finely, chopped onion
¼ cup shredded carrot
¼ tsp fine herbs
1/8 tsp pepper

Thaw fish if frozen. Cut into 8 portions

Trim the large center vein from each cabbage leaf, keeping leaf in one piece.

Rinse leaves and place in a 12+7 ½ + 2- inch baking dish. Cover with vented clear plastic wrap. Cook on high 100% power for 3 to 5 minutes or till tender.

In a 1- quart casserole stir together the shredded cabbage, zucchini, onion and carrot. Cook covered, on high 3 to 5 minutes or till tender, stirring once.

Drain. Stir in fine herbs and pepper.

Spoon some of the vegetable mixture atop the center of each piece of fish.

Bring the ends of the fish up around the filling. Place fish roll near one end of a cabbage leaf. Fold in two sides of the leaf; then roll up beginning from an unfolded end. Secure with toothpicks, if necessary.

Place seam side down in the baking dish. Repeat with remaining fish and cabbage leaves.

Cook covered on high 4to 6 minutes or till fish flakes easily with a fork, giving dish a half turn once.

Makes 4 servings
Each serving provides= 1 protein 1 vegetable

Enjoy!

ORANGE ROUGHY IN CITRUS SAUCE

Ingredients

1 pound orange Roughy
¼ cup frozen orange concentrate
2 tbsp. lemon juice
1 tsp dried dill weed
1 tsp paprika
2 tbsp. minced fresh parsley or 1 tbsp. dried
½ cup water
3 tbsp. + 3 tbsp. fruit juice sweetened orange marmalade
1 tsp arrowroot

Directions

Place fish in shallow non- metal casserole.

Combine remaining ingredients except marmalade and arrowroot and mix to dissolve orange juice concentrate. Reserve ½ cup for sauce pour remaining mixture over fish. Cover fish and marinate in refrigerator for 45 minutes or longer, turning at least once.

Preheat broiler

Remove fish from marinade and place on broiler pan. Add 3 tbsp. of marmalade to marinade and heat. Broil fish 4- inches from heat 10 to 15 minutes, until fish flakes, basting with marinade several times during cooking.

While fish is broiling, heat reserved orange sauce in small saucepan with arrowroot and remaining 3 tbsp. marmalade until sauce begins to thicken.

Transfer fish to serving dish. Pour sauce on fish or serve on side. If desired, decorate the plate with fresh oranges slices and sprigs of parsley.

Makes 4 servings
Each serving provides 1 protein 1 fat

Enjoy!

POACHED FISH DINNER WITH MUSTARD- DILL SAUCE

Ingredients

4 medium thin skinned potatoes cut in ¼ inch slices (about 3 cups)
2 medium zucchini, cut into ¼ inch rounds (about 2 cups)
2 medium carrots cut into ¼ inch rounds (about 1 cup)
3 cups water
3 tbsp. lemon juice
1 inch strip lemon peel
2 slices onion
4 sprigs parsley
1 bay leaf
¾ lb halibut (1 inch thick)
1 cup mustard dill sauce

Directions:

Steam potatoes and carrots for 15 minutes; add Zucchini and steam for additional 10 minutes or until desired texture is reached.

Bring poaching ingredients (water, lemon peel, onion, parsley and bay leaf) to boil in a broad shallow pan or skillet, simmer 5-10 minutes to extract flavor from seasoning.

Add fish. Simmer, partially covered, 10 minutes, or until fish flakes with a fork.

Remove fish with a slotted spatula and drain. Place on serving plate, surround with potatoes and vegetables.

Spoon mustard-dill sauce over all; serve any remaining sauce on the table.

Makes 4 servings
Each serving provides = 1 protein, 1 starch, 1 fat, 1 veg.

Enjoy!

OVEN FRIED FISH

Ingredients

2 cups no salt, crackers, processed to fine crumbs
¼ tsp dry mustard powder
1 egg white
2 tbsp. milk
1 pound white fish filets your choice
Lemon wedges (optional)

Directions:

Preheat oven to 425%F

Process crackers into fine crumbs using food processor or blender stir dry mustard into crumbs. Beat egg white with milk in a broad shallow bowl.

Spread cracker crumbs on a plate; dip fish filets one at a time into egg white mixture, then place in cracker crumbs and turn to coat all surfaces.

Place on baking sheet and bake at 425% F. for about 15 minutes until coating is crisp and fish flakes easily with a fork.

Serve with lemon wedges, if desired
Makes 4 servings; each serving provides= 1 protein, ½ starch

Enjoy!

COUSCOUS WITH RAISINS DATES AND CURRY

Ingredients

1 ½ cups chicken stock
¾ cup couscous
1 tbsp. margarine
¾ cup finely chopped onions
1 tsp crushed garlic
1 cup finely chopped red pepper
¼ cup raisins
1 tsp curry powder
5 dried dates or apricots, chopped

In a small saucepan, bring chicken stock to a boil. Stir in couscous and remove from heat. Cover and let stand until liquid is absorbed, 5 to 8 minutes. Place in serving bowl. Meanwhile in non-stick saucepan, melt margarine sauté' onions, garlic and red pepper until softened, approximately 5 minutes. Add raisins, curry powder and dates; mix until combined. Add to couscous and mix well.

Makes 4 servings = ½ cup. Each serving provides = 1 starch, 1 fat. Enjoy!

FISH FILETS

Ingredients

1lb orange Roughy filets or other mild white fish
½ cup plain yogurt
2 tbsp. frozen orange concentrate
1 tbsp. lemon juice
2 tsp marmalade
1/3 cup mashed banana
1/8 tsp garlic powder
½ tsp ground ginger
Pinch white pepper (optional)

Directions:

Preheat oven to 400%F.

Cut filets into 4 serving size pieces, place side by side in baking pan large enough to hold fish in a single layer.

In a medium bowl, combine rest of ingredients; pour ½ cup mixture evenly over fish.

Bake 10 to 15 minutes or until fish flakes. Timing will vary depending on thickness of filets.

Remove fish from pan, place on serving dish and serve with remaining sauce.

Makes 4 servings
Each serving provides 1 protein, 1 fat.

Enjoy!

APRICOT CHICKEN

Ingredients

2 cups canned apricots, packed solid
4 skinless chicken breasts
1 large onion, chopped coarsely ground black pepper to taste
2 sage leaves, finely chopped or ½ tsp dried sage
1 sprig thyme, chopped
1 tbsp. fruit chutney
1 tbsp. cornstarch
2 tbsp. water

GARNISH:

4 apricot halves reserved from main quantity
1 tbsp. finely chopped chives or mint

Reserve 4 apricot halves for garnish.

Puree remaining apricots in a food processor or blender or press through a sieve.

Arrange chicken fillets in a single layer in a casserole. Sprinkle with onion, pepper and herbs.

Combine chutney and apricot puree and pour over the chicken.

Bake for 30 minutes.

Mix the cornstarch and water to a smooth paste.

Remove casserole from oven. Use a slotted spoon to lift out chicken breasts; cover and keep warm.

Drain the sauce from the casserole into a saucepan. Add the cornstarch paste to the sauce and heat, stirring constantly, until it thickens. Cook a further 2 minutes.

Arrange a chicken breast on each plate and spoon sauce over each one.

Garnish with the reserved apricot halves and sprinkle with chopped chives.

Prep time =40 minutes

Oven temp 350%F.

Each serving provides = 1 protein, 1 fruit

Enjoy!

SWEET AND SOUR CHICKEN

Ingredients

1 cup pineapple chunks canned in juice
2 tbsp. arrowroot
3 tbsp. apple cider vinegar
3-4 tbsp. honey
1 tsp mustard, spicy or Dijon
2 tsp ketchup
Dash cayenne pepper (optional)
¼ cup chicken stock
¾ tsp powdered ginger
1 large onion cut in crescents
2 cloves garlic, chopped
1 cup quartered mushrooms
1 green pepper; cut in 1- ½ -inch strips
¾ lb boned, skinless chicken breast meat, cut into 1-inch pieces
¼ lb snow peas, ends trimmed
1 tomato; cut in bite – sized pieces

Drain pineapple and reserve ½ cup juice. Mix juice with arrowroot, vinegar, honey, mustard, ketchup and cayenne and set aside.

Heat 2 to 4 tablespoons broth in wok or large skillet: Stir-fry ginger, onion, garlic, mushrooms, green pepper and chicken for about 10 minutes, until chicken is cooked. Pour off any accumulated liquid.

Stir juice mixture, and pour into pan along with pineapple chunks, snow peas and tomatoes. Stir over medium heat 3 to 5 minutes, until sauce thickens. Remove from heat and serve.

Makes 4 servings
Each serving provides = 1 protein, 1 vegetable, 1 fat

Enjoy!

PORK ROAST

Ingredients

1 boneless pork top loin roast (3 pounds)
2 cloves garlic, thinly sliced
2 tbsp. Dijon mustard
1 tsp red wine vinegar
¾ tsp ground thyme
½ tsp ground sage
¾ cup beef stock
¾ cup unsweetened apple juice
¼ cup apricot jam
1 ½ cups peeled and chopped Granny Smith apples
1 tbsp. sour cream
1 tbsp. cornstarch

Cut 8 deep slits in the top of roast using a very sharp knife. Insert garlic into slits.

Mix mustard, vinegar, thyme and sage in a small bowl. Using a pastry brush, coat roast with all of the mustard mixture, place roast in roasting pan.

Warm the stock, apple juice and jam in a small saucepan over medium-high heat until jam melts. Pour over roast. Arrange chopped apples around roast. Cover,

Roast at; 350%F. for 1 ¼ to 1 ½ hours, basting every 30 minutes or so.

Remove roast from pan and keep warm. Reserve ½ cup pan juices; pour remaining pan juices and apples into a medium saucepan. Skim off as much fat as possible.

Into reserved ½ cup pan juices, add sour cream and mix well, add cornstarch and blend again until smooth.

Bring pan juices and apples (in a saucepan) to a boil. Whisk in sour cream mixture and cook over medium – high heat for 2 minutes, until bubbly and thickened. Serve apple gravy over thin slices of pork.

Makes 8 servings
Each serving provides= 1 protein, 1 fruit, 1 fat

Enjoy!

MEATLOAF TOPPED WITH SAUTEED VEGETABLES AND TOMATO SAUCE

Preheat oven to 375%F.
9+5-inch loaf pan sprayed with pam

Sauce Ingredients
1 ½ tsp vegetable oil
1 tsp crushed garlic
½ cup finely diced onions
½ cup finely diced sweet red pepper
½ cup thinly sliced mushrooms
½ cup tomato sauce, heated

Meatloaf ingredients
1 lb ground beef, chicken or turkey
1 green onion, finely chopped
2 tsp crushed garlic
1 egg
1/3 cup dry bread crumbs
2 tbsp. chili sauce
½ tsp dried basil
½ tsp dried oregano
½ cup tomato sauce

Meatloaf: In bowl, mix together beef, onion, garlic, egg, bread crumbs, chili sauce, basil, oregano and tomato sauce until well combined. Pat into loaf pan.

In small non-stick skillet, heat oil; sauté garlic, onions, red pepper and mushrooms until softened, about 5 minutes. Spoon over meatloaf; bake uncovered, for 40 to 50 minutes or until meat thermometer registers 170%F.

Cover and let stand for 20 minutes before serving. Serve with tomato sauce.

Makes 6 servings
Each serving provides = 1 protein, 1 ½ vegetables, 1 fat, 1/3 starch

Enjoy!

VEGETABLE CURRY

Ingredients

1 lb mixed vegetables
2 tsp olive oil
1 onion, sliced
1 tsp turmeric
½ tsp ground cumin
¾ inch piece green ginger, chopped
1 or 2 fresh hot chillies or chili powder to taste
1 cup water
1 cup coconut milk
1 tbsp. lemon juice

Trim vegetables and cut into pieces. Heat oil until very hot: in wok or large frying pan. Add onion and spices and toss until onion is golden brown. Add the rest of the vegetables and stir fry for 2 to 3 minutes Add 1 cup water and cook 6 to 8 minutes, uncovered, or until vegetables are tender. Add coconut milk and bring to a boil. Remove from heat. Add lemon juice. Serve with brown rice.

Makes 4 servings
Each serving provides = 1 ½ vegetables, 1 fat

Enjoy!

FIVE -SPICE CHICKEN

Ingredients

¼ tsp Chinese five – spice powder
½ tsp chili powder
1 clove garlic, crushed
¾ cup plain yogurt
4 skinless chicken breasts

Fold five- spice powder, chili powder, soy sauce and garlic gently into yogurt

Coat chicken breasts in yogurt mixture and let it marinate at least 4 hours.

Place in shallow casserole, cover with lid or aluminum foil and bake for 1 hour in a low to moderate oven or until tender, turning occasionally.

Prep time 1 ¼ hours: plus 4 hours marinating time. Oven temp 300%F.

Cooking equipment: shallow casserole or baking dish

Makes 4 servings: Each serving provides 1 protein

Enjoy!

VEGETARIAN LASAGNA

Sauce: ingredients

Oil
2 med onions peeled and chopped
3 large tomatoes
5oz tomato paste
2 cups water
1 to 2 tsp crushed or finely chopped garlic
1 tsp dried mixed herbs
¼ tsp black pepper
26oz can three bean mix or kidney beans

LAYERS:

8oz frozen spinach
9 sheets instant spinach or whole wheat lasagne noodles
1 cup cottage cheese
2 tbsp. grated parmesan cheese

Wipe a large frying pan with oil. Heat it and sauté onions in frying pan until lightly browned, stirring to prevent burning. Add tomatoes and cook for about 5 minutes, until soft. Add tomato paste and water and mix thoroughly. Add seasonings. Rinse and drain beans and add to frying pan. Combine well. Simmer gently, covered, until you are ready to assemble the lasagne. If sauce becomes too thick, add a little water.

To assemble:

Spoon a thin layer of tomato and bean sauce over base of lasagna dish. Arrange a layer of noodles on top. Spoon on more sauce, sprinkle with half the cottage cheese. Top with another layer of noodles and cover this with spinach and cottage cheese. Place the last layer of noodles over this, cover with remaining sauce and, lastly sprinkle with parmesan cheese.

Cover with foil and bake for 30 minutes at 350%F. remove the foil, and bake for a further 30 minutes or until noodles are tender.

Makes 6 servings
Each serving provides = 1 starch, 1 vegetable, 1 protein

Enjoy!

SPINACH /MUSHROOM LASAGNA

Ingredients

2/3 cup chopped onion
4 cloves garlic, chopped
2-3 tbsp. chicken stock
2 cups sliced mushrooms
2 cans (15oz each) no salt tomatoes
3 tbsp. honey
2 tsp crushed dried oregano
1 tsp crushed dried basil
Pinch white pepper (optional)
10oz package frozen chopped spinach thawed and well drained
2 cups cottage cheese
4 egg whites, lightly beaten
1 ½ tsp Italian seasoning blend
9 whole wheat lasagna noodles, uncooked

DIRECTIONS:

In a medium saucepan, cook onion and garlic in chicken stock for 3 minutes, until softened and beginning to color, over med high heat. Add mushrooms and cook, stirring constantly, until they soften and release their juices.

To above mixture add tomato sauce, honey, oregano, basil and white pepper. Bring to a boil and simmer gently 5 to 10 minutes to blend flavors.

Preheat oven to 350%F.

Press as much moisture as possible from thawed frozen spinach. Combine with cottage cheese, egg whites and Italian seasoning blend.

Spread ½ cup sauce over bottom of an 8-inch baking pan. Cover with 1/3 of the noodles (break noodles to fit 8-inch pan) add 1 ¼ cups sauce and half the cottage cheese mixture.

Repeat this layering with noodles, 1 ¼ cups sauce and remaining cottage cheese mixture. Top with remaining noodles. Spread remaining sauce (about 1 cup) over top of lasagna. Cover pan and bake at 350%F. 1 hour. Remove cover and bake 15-30 minutes longer, until pasta is tender.

Makes 6 servings
Each serving provides = 1 starch, 1 vegetable, ½ fat, ½ protein

Enjoy!

BEEF STEW

Ingredients

1 ½ pounds boneless top sirloin
2 cups sliced leeks
2 cloves garlic, minced
2 ½ cups beef stock
1 whole clove
1 bay leaf
3 cups each chopped carrots and sliced mushrooms
3 cups peeled, cubed potatoes
1 tsp ground thyme
1/3 cup tomato based chili sauce
1 cup water or (light beer optional)
2 tbsp. cornstarch
¼ cup chopped fresh parsley
½ tsp black pepper

Spray a large saucepan with pam. Add beef cubes and cook over medium –high heat until no longer pink, about 10 minutes. Add leeks and garlic.

Cook and stir for 5 minutes. Stir in ½ cup of beef stock. Reduce heat to medium and cook, uncovered, until liquid has evaporated, about 15 minutes. Stir occasionally.

Stir in remaining beef broth, clove and bay leaf. Bring to a boil. Reduce heat to medium – low. Cover and simmer for 40 minutes (stir every once in a while).

Add carrots, mushrooms, potatoes and thyme. Stir well. Cover and simmer another 40 minutes, until vegetables and meat are tender.

Stir in chili sauce. Combine water or beer and cornstarch in a small bowl. Add to stew. Cook and stir until sauce thickens, 1-2 minutes. Stir in parsley and pepper.

Remove bay leaf and serve immediately.

Makes 6 servings
Each serving provides = 1 protein, 1 vegetable, 1 starch, 1 fat

Enjoy!

INDIAN LAMB IN SPINACH SAUCE

Ingredients

6 ripe tomatoes
1 tbsp. olive oil
2 cloves garlic, finely chopped
2 tsp fresh ginger, finely chopped
2 fresh green or red chilies, finely chopped
Sea salt to taste
1 lb lamb, diced
¼ tsp each of ground cumin, coriander, cinnamon, cloves and turmeric
3 bunches fresh spinach, finely chopped, or 1.5lb frozen spinach thawed

Blend tomatoes in food processor or blender. Heat oil in saucepan, add garlic, ginger, chilies, and sea salt, cook stirring for 2 minutes. Add lamb, mix well, cover and cook over low heat for 30 to 40 minutes or until lamb is tender. Add tomatoes and cook for a further 10 minutes. Add spices and simmer gently for 10 minutes. Add spinach and simmer for a further 4 minutes.

Makes 4 to 5 servings
Each serving provides = 1 protein, 2 vegetables, ¾ fat

Enjoy!

MOGUL LAMB

Ingredients: heat oven to 350%F.

6 large ripe tomatoes
½ cup water
4 cloves garlic, finely chopped
2 tsp ginger, finely chopped
3 fresh chillies, finely chopped
1 tsp ground black pepper, ½ tsp each ground cardamom, cloves, fennel, cinnamon, and fenugreek. 4 tbsp. fresh coriander leaves, chopped
1 tbsp. each, fresh basil, dill and mint chopped. Sea salt to taste
3lb lamb, boned and trimmed of all visible fat

Place tomatoes, garlic, ginger, chillies and pepper into a saucepan and simmer, stirring occasionally for 15 minutes. Add all other ingredients, but the lamb, mix well and set aside. Place the lamb into a casserole dish, cover well with tomato mixture, cover and let stand for 20 minutes in the refrigerator to marinate. Place uncovered in oven and bake for 1 ½ hours or until cooked. Makes 6 to 8 servings= each serving provides 1 protein, 1 veg, 1 fat

Enjoy!

MICROWAVE MAIN DISH
CHICKEN OR TURKEY WITH MUSHROOMS

Ingredients

2 cups sliced fresh mushrooms
¼ cup chicken stock
1 clove garlic, minced
¼ tsp dried basil, crushed
2 cups cubed chicken or turkey (11 ounces)
14oz can artichoke hearts, drained and cut into wedged
1 cup milk
3 tbsp. flour
1/8 tsp sea salt
Dash pepper
1 tbsp. snipped fresh parsley

In a 2-quart casserole combine mushrooms, chicken stock, garlic and basil. Cook, covered on 100% power (high) for 3 to 4 minutes or until mushrooms are tender, stirring once. Stir in chicken and artichoke hearts. In a small bowl stir together milk, flour, salt and pepper. Stir into casserole. Cooked uncovered; on high for 6 to 9 minutes or until thickened and bubbly: Stirring after every minute. Cook 1 minute more. Sprinkle with parsley.

Makes 4 servings
Each serving provides = 1 protein, 1 vegetable, 1 fat

Enjoy!

MICROWAVE MAIN DISH
SWEET & SOUR FISH

Ingredients

1pound fresh or frozen fish steaks
1 medium green or sweet red pepper, cut into one inch squared (1 cup)
1 medium carrot, thinly sliced (½ cup)
½ cup chicken stock
1 clove garlic, minced
2 tbsp. brown sugar
4 tsp cornstarch
2 tbsp. vinegar
2 tbsp. soy sauce
½ cup seedless grapes, halved

Cut fish into ¾ -inch pieces

In a 1 ½ - quart casserole dish cook fish on 100% power (high) for 3 to 5 minutes until fish flakes easily when tested with a fork, stirring once. Drain; set aside.

In the casserole combine pepper, carrot, chicken stock and garlic. Cook, covered, on high for 3 to 5 minutes or until vegetables are just crisp-tender, stirring once. Do not drain.

In a small mixing bowl stir together brown sugar, cornstarch, vinegar and soy sauce. Stir into vegetable mixture. Cook uncovered on high for 1 to 2 minutes or until thickened and bubbly, stirring every 30 seconds.

Gently stir in fish and grapes. Cook uncovered, for 1 minute more or until heated through. If desired, serve with hot cooked rice.

Makes 4 servings
Each serving provides 1 protein 1 fat 1 vegetable

Enjoy!

MICROWAVE MAIN DISH
FISH STEAKS WITH MUSHROOM SAUCE

Ingredients

4-4-ounce fresh or fresh or frozen halibut or other fish steaks, cut ¾ inches thick
2 tsp cornstarch
½ tsp instant chicken bouillon granules
½ cup milk
1 cup mushrooms, sliced
¼ cup shredded carrot
½ tsp finely shredded lemon peel
1 tbsp. snipped fresh parsley

Thaw fish, if frozen

Arrange fish steaks in an 8+8+2- inch baking dish. Cover with vented clear plastic wrap. Cook on 100% power (high) for 4 to 8 minutes or until fish flakes easily when tested with a fork. Keep warm while preparing sauce.

In a 2- cup measure stir together cornstarch and bouillon granules. Stir in milk all at once. Cook uncovered; on high for 1 ½ to 3 minutes or until thickened and bubbly; stirring after 1 minute, then every 30 seconds.

Stir in mushrooms and carrot. Cook for 30 to 60 seconds more until heated through. Stir in lemon peel. Serve over fish steaks. Sprinkle with parsley.

Makes 4 servings
Each serving provides = 1 protein ¾ vegetable 1 fat

Enjoy!

MICROWAVE MAIN DISH
STEAMED SOLE IN CABBAGE

Ingredients

1 pound fresh sole or other fish fillets
8 medium cabbage leaves or savoy cabbage
¾ cup shredded cabbage
½ cup shredded zucchini
1/3 cup finely, chopped onion
¼ cup shredded carrot
¼ tsp fine herbs
1/8 tsp pepper

Thaw fish if frozen. Cut into 8 portions.

Trim the large center vein from each cabbage leaf, keeping the leaf in one piece.

Rinse leaves and place in a 12+7+2-inch baking dish. Cover with vented clear plastic wrap. Cook on high 100% power for 3 to 5 minutes or until tender.

In a 1- quart casserole stir together the shredded cabbage, zucchini, onion and carrot. Cook covered, on high 3 to 5 minutes or until tender, stirring once.

Drain. Stir in fine herbs and pepper.

Spoon some of the vegetable mixture atop the center of each piece of fish.

Bring the ends of the fish up around the filling. Place fish roll near one end of a cabbage leaf. Fold in two sides of the leaf, and roll up beginning from an unfolded end. Secure with toothpicks, if necessary. Place seam side down in the baking dish. Repeat with remaining fish and cabbage leaves.

Cook covered on high 4 to 6 minutes or until fish flakes easily with a fork, giving dish a half turn once.

Makes 4 servings
Each serving provides = 1 protein 1 vegetable

Enjoy!

MICROWAVE MAIN DISH
SPINACH- STUFFED SOLE

Ingredients

4 fresh or frozen sole fillets (about ¾ pound total)
1 Egg white, beaten
1 cup herb- seasoned croutons
½ cup cottage cheese
¼ cup shredded carrot
2 tbsp. cocktail sauce
10 ounce package frozen chopped spinach, thawed and well drained
Non-stick spray coating

Thaw fish, if frozen.

For stuffing, in a mixing bowl stir together egg white, croutons, cottage cheese, carrot and cocktail sauce. Stir in the drained spinach.

Spray four 10- ounce custard cups with non-stick spray coating. Line cups with fish fillets, trimming and piecing if necessary.

Spoon stuffing into the center of each cup; arrange filled cups in the microwave. Cover loosely with waxed paper. Cook on high for 5 to 6 minutes or until fish flakes easily when tested with a fork and stuffing is heated through. Rotate and rearrange the cups once during cooking.

To serve, slide the fish and stuffing out of the custard cups onto individual serving plates.

Makes 4 servings
Each serving provides = 1 protein 1 vegetable 1 fat ½ starch

Enjoy!

FISH CAKES

Ingredients

1 cup cereal
¼ cup chicken stock
1 can 6 ½ ounces light tuna or pink salmon, packed in water, rinsed and drained
Dash white pepper (optional)
1 tsp onion powder
1 egg white
1 tsp prepared mustard, spicy or Dijon

Directions:

Preheat oven to 375%F. or preheat broiler if broiling is preferred

Combine cereal and stock in small saucepan and cook for 3 minutes stirring occasionally, until mixture thickens

Remove cereal mixture from heat and add fish, pepper, onion powder, egg white and mustard, mashing with a fork until well blended.

When cool enough to handle, shape into 4 patties on a baking sheet.

To bake, place in oven for 10 minutes; turn patties over and bake 5 minutes longer.

If you prefer to broil, place about 5-inches beneath heat and broil 5 minutes on each side, until nicely browned.

Makes 2 servings
Each serving provides = 1 protein 1 starch ½ fat

Enjoy!

MICROWAVE MAIN DISH
SPINACH STUFFED FLANK STEAK

Ingredients

10 ounce package frozen chopped spinach
½ cup chopped onion
½ cup shredded carrot
1 clove garlic, minced
¼ tsp dried basil, crushed
1lb beef flank steak
¼ tsp pepper
¼ tsp sea salt

In a 1 ½ - quart casserole combine spinach, onion, carrot and garlic; cook covered, on 100% power (high) 6-7 minutes or until vegetables are tender stirring twice.

Drain well, squeezing out excess moisture. Stir in basil.

Meanwhile, use a sharp knife to score one side of the steak.

Place meat, scored side up between 2 sheets of plastic wrap.

Pound meat to ½ inch thickness: Sprinkle with salt and pepper.

Spoon spinach mixture over meat; roll up from one long side.

Secure with wooden picks at even intervals, beginning ¾ inch from one end.

Cut between picks into 6 slices.

Place meat rolls, cut side up, in a 12+7 ½ + 2 – inch baking dish.

Flatten slightly with your hand. Cover with wax paper.

Cook on 100% power (high) for 5 minutes. Rearrange meat and spoon juices over. Cook on 50% (medium) for 10 to 15 minutes or until meat is tender, rearranging once. Remove wooden picks and serve meat with juices

Makes 6 servings
Each serving provides = 1 protein 1 fat ½ veg

Enjoy!

MICROWAVE MAIN DISH ORIENTAL BEEF AND BROCCOLI

Ingredients

¾ lb beef top round steak
1 tbsp. soy sauce
1 tbsp. vinegar
1 tbsp. molasses
1 clove garlic, minced
¼ tsp crushed red pepper
1 cup thinly sliced carrots
6 cups fresh broccoli
1 ½ tsp cornstarch
1 tbsp. water

Thinly slice meat across the grain into bite size strips: Set-aside.

In a 2- quart casserole dish stir together soy sauce, vinegar, molasses, garlic and red pepper. Stir in meat. Cover and let stand at room temperature for 10 minutes.

Cook meat mixture, covered at 100% power (high) for 3 to 5 minutes or until meat is no longer pink, stirring every 2 minutes.

With a slotted spoon, remove meat from casserole; set aside. Reserve juices in casserole: add carrots to juices in casserole. Cook, covered on high for 1 minute. Add broccoli and cook 4 to 6 minutes more until vegetables are nearly crisp- tender, stirring every 2 minutes.

Stir together cornstarch and water; stir into vegetables: cook uncovered, on high for 2 to 3 minutes or until slightly thickened, stirring after every minute.

Stir in meat, cook covered on high for 1 minute or until heated through.

Makes 4 servings
Each serving provides = 1 protein 1 fat 1 ½ vegetables

Enjoy!

MICROWAVE MAIN DISH
LEMONY TURKEY MEATBALLS

Ingredients

1 egg white, beaten
¼ cup whole bran cereal or rolled oats
1 tsp Worcestershire sauce
½ tsp finely shredded lemon peal
1 pound ground raw turkey
1 cup chicken stock
1 cup broccoli flowerets
½ cup thinly sliced carrots
1 green onion, sliced
¼ cup plain yogurt
1 tbsp. cornstarch
1 tsp lemon juice
3 cups hot cooked noodles

In a mixing bowl combine egg white, cereal, Worcestershire sauce, and lemon peel. Add turkey; mix well (mixture will be soft). Shape into 24 meatballs.

Arrange meatballs in a 12+7 ½ + 2-inch dish. Cover with wax paper. Cook on 100% power (high) for 4 to 6 minutes or until meatballs are no longer pink, rearranging and turning meatballs over after 3 minutes. Drain off fat.

Meanwhile, for sauce, in a 4 cup measure stir together chicken stock, broccoli, carrot and green onion. In a small bowl stir together yogurt and cornstarch; stir into vegetable mixture.

Cook sauce, uncovered on high for 4 to 6 minutes or until thickened and bubbly, stirring after every minute until slightly thickened, then every 30 seconds. Stir in lemon juice; pour over meatballs.

Serve over noodles.

Makes 6 servings
Each serving provides = 1 protein 1 fat 1 starch 1 vegetable

Enjoy!

PASTA PRIMAVERA

Ingredients

2 cups whole button mushrooms
2 cups cubed zucchini (cut into 1- inch cubes)
2 cups coarsely chopped tomatoes
1 cup each, sliced sweet red and yellow peppers
1 tbsp. olive oil
2 cloves; garlic minced
3 tbsp. chopped fresh basil or 1 ½ tsp dried basil
¼ tsp freshly ground pepper
12oz uncooked tri-color rotini (about 4 cups dry)
1 ½ cups broccoli florets
½ cup frozen peas, thawed
2 tbsp. each: parmesan cheese and chopped fresh parsley

Preheat oven to 400%F.
Spray a 13+9- inch baking pan with non-stick spray. Set aside.

In a large bowl, combine mushrooms, zucchini, tomatoes, sweet peppers, olive oil, garlic, basil and pepper. Toss until vegetables are evenly coated with oil and seasonings. Transfer vegetables to prepared baking pan. Bake uncovered, for 25 minutes. Stir once, halfway through cooking time.

Meanwhile, prepare pasta according to package directions. About 4 minutes before pasta is ready, add broccoli and peas to the boiling water. When pasta is cooked, drain pasta and vegetables, then return them to the pot. Stir in roasted vegetables, parmesan cheese and parsley.

Serve with extra freshly ground black pepper, if desired.

Makes 4 servings
Each serving provides = 2 vegetables, 1 starch, ½ fat, ¼ protein

Enjoy!

GADO- GADO

Ingredients

1 cup bean sprouts
1 cup green beans
1 ½ cups broccoli florets
1 cup sliced carrots
1 cup diced cabbage
1 medium green bell pepper sliced
6-10 snow peas
2 tomatoes cut into wedges
2 onions cut into wedges
1 small cucumber, peeled and diced
2 eggs hard boiled, cut into quarters

You have free range with this recipe to add or to change vegetables according to season or taste.

Half fill a medium saucepan with water and bring to a rapid boil. Plunge the vegetables, except the tomatoes and cucumber, one variety at a time, into the boiling water for no more than 1 minute, or until the color intensifies, or microwave with 2 tbsp. water on high for 2 minutes. Quickly remove the blanched vegetables from the water, place in a colander and immediately rinse with cold, running water; this preserves the color and crispness.

Bring water back to boil before blanching each type of vegetable.

Arrange all the ingredients on a platter.

Serve as an appetizer or entrée at either room temperature or chilled with cooked brown rice and a dish of warm sate' (peanut) sauce.

To store: cover and refrigerate for no more than one day

Makes 4 servings
Each serving provides = 2 vegetables, ½ protein

Enjoy!

BROAD BEAN & SMOKED SALMON SALAD

Ingredients

8oz fava or Lima beans, fresh or frozen
3oz smoked salmon, thinly sliced
12 cherry tomatoes
1 small white onion, thinly sliced
2 tbsp. lemon juice
2 tsp olive oil
2 tsp capers, drained
2 tsp chopped fresh parsley

Cook beans until they are soft, but still retain their shape

Combine cooked beans, smoked salmon, cherry tomatoes and white onion in a bowl.

Blend all the other ingredients in a screw top jar and pour over the salad

Chill and serve.

Makes 4 servings

Each serving provides = 1 protein, ¼ vegetable, ½ fat

Enjoy!

MEATLESS MAIN DISH
TOFU AND VEGETABLE STIR FRY

Ingredients

½ cup water
¼ cup dry sherry
1 tbsp. cornstarch
2 tbsp. soy sauce
1 tsp sugar
1 tsp instant chicken bouillon granules
¾ tsp ground ginger
Non -stick spray coating
1 cup thinly sliced carrots
1 clove garlic, minced
3 cups broccoli, cut up
6oz tofu, cubed
1 cup hot cooked brown rice

For sauce; stir together the water, dry sherry, cornstarch, soy sauce, sugar, bouillon granules and ginger. Set aside.

Spray wok or large skillet with non- stick spray coating. Preheat over medium – high heat.

Add carrots and garlic and stir fry for 2 minutes. Add broccoli and stir fry for 3 to 4 minutes more or until all vegetables are crisp – tender. Push vegetables from center of wok.

Stir sauce and add to center of wok. Cook and stir until thickened and bubbly.

Add tofu to wok. Stir ingredients together to coat with sauce.

Cook and stir for 1 minute serve with hot cooked rice.

Makes 4 servings
Each serving provides = 1 protein, 1 vegetable, 1 starch

Enjoy!

CHICKEN CACCIATORE

Ingredients

1 (15oz can) no salt tomatoes in juice, cut up and thoroughly drained
1 cup no salt tomato sauce
1 ½ tsp crushed dried oregano
½ tsp crushed dried basil
1 tbsp. honey
¼ tsp white pepper
¼ cup chicken stock
3 cloves garlic, chopped
1 cup chopped onion
1 large green pepper cut in 1 inch strips
¾ lb boned, skinless, chicken breast meat, cut in 2-inch cubes
¾ cup frozen green peas
1 tbsp. balsamic vinegar

Place cut up canned tomatoes that have been thoroughly drained, tomato sauce, oregano, basil, honey and pepper in a 2-3 quart saucepan cover and simmer 15 minutes.

Heat 4 tbsp. broth in a large skillet: over medium – high heat. Stir fry garlic, onion, green pepper and chicken for about 10 minutes, until chicken is no longer pink inside.

Add chicken and green peppers to sauce and simmer, partially covered, 10 minutes. Add peas and balsamic vinegar, and cook uncovered an additional 5 minutes.

Makes 4 servings = 1 cup
Each serving provides = 1 protein, 1 vegetable, 1 fat

Enjoy!

CHINESE BEEF WITH CHRISP VEGETABLES

Ingredients

1 tbsp. vegetable oil
2 tsp crushed garlic
8oz lean beef, thinly sliced
1 ½ cups chopped broccoli
1 ½ cups thinly sliced sweet red pepper
1 ½ cups snow peas

Ingredients for sauce

1 tbsp. cornstarch
¾ cup beef stock
2 tbsp. soya sauce
¼ cup brown sugar
2 tbsp. rice vinegar
1 ½ tsp minced gingerroot or ¼ tsp ground

Sauce: in a small bowl, combine cornstarch, beef stock, soya sauce, sugar, sherry and ginger; mix well and set aside.

In a large non-stick skillet, heat oil; sauté garlic and beef just until beef is browned but not cooked through. Remove beef and set aside.

To skillet, add broccoli, red pepper and snow peas; sauté for 2 minutes return beef to pan. Stir sauce and add to pan; cook just until beef is cooked and sauce has thickened, approximately 2 minutes, stirring constantly.

Makes 4 servings
Each serving provides = 1 protein, 1 vegetable, 1 fat

Enjoy!

SWEET POTATO, APPLE AND RAISIN CASSERLOE

Preheat oven to 350%F.
Baking dish sprayed with pam

Ingredients

1 lb sweet potatoes, peeled and cubed
¾ tsp ground ginger
¼ cup honey
¾ tsp ground cinnamon
2 tbsp. margarine, melted
¼ cup raisins
2 tbsp. chopped walnuts
¾ cup cubed peeled sweet apples

Steam or microwave sweet potatoes: just until slightly underdone.
Drain and place in baking dish

In a small bowl, combine ginger, honey, cinnamon, margarine, raisins, walnuts and apples; mix well.

Pour over sweet potatoes and bake uncovered, for 20 minutes or until tender.

Makes 6 servings
Each serving provides = 1 starch, 1 fat, ½ fruit

Enjoy!

SHEPHERD'S PIE

Ingredients

4 medium potatoes, peeled and quartered
½ cup milk or buttermilk
½ tsp sea salt
1 lb lean ground beef
¼ cup unseasoned dry bread crumbs
¼ cup minced onion
1 egg
1 tbsp. ketchup
1 clove garlic, minced
¼ tsp black pepper
1 large tomato, thinly sliced
½ tsp dried, oregano
¼ cup shredded Swiss cheese (1 ounce)
¼ cup crumbled feta cheese (1 ounce)
½ 10oz package frozen spinach, thawed, squeezed dry and chopped (5oz total)

Cook potatoes in a large pot of boiling water until tender, about 20 minutes. Drain well. Add milk and salt. Mash until smooth. Set aside.

In a large bowl, combine beef, breadcrumbs, onions, egg, ketchup, garlic and black pepper. Mix well (using your hands works best).

Pat beef mixture over bottom and up the sides of a 9 inch pie plate.

Layer tomato slices over beef. Sprinkle oregano over tomatoes. Spread Swiss and feta cheeses over tomatoes. Put spinach on top of cheese. Spoon mashed potatoes over spinach. Spread evenly, leaving a 1- inch border around edges. Meat and potatoes should not touch. Smooth top.

Bake at 350%F. for 45 minutes. Let cool 5 minutes. Slice into wedges and serve.

Try it with ground turkey instead of beef.

Makes 6 servings
Each serving provides = 1 protein, 1 starch, 1 fat

Enjoy!

MICROWAVE MAIN DISH
TEX-MEX TURKEY TENDERLOINS

Ingredients

Four 4ounce turkey tenderloin steaks, about ½ inch thick
1 tsp ground Cumin
1/8 tsp pepper
1 tbsp. sugar
2 tbsp. vinegar
1 ½ tsp cornstarch
1 large tomato, seeded and chopped
1 cup zucchini
¼ cup sliced green onions
4oz diced green chili peppers
2 cups hot cooked rice

Rinse turkey steaks; pat dry. Stir together cumin and pepper; sprinkle on both sides of the turkey steaks.

In a 12+7 ½ +2- inch dish arrange the turkey with meaty portions toward the edges of the dish.

Cover with vented microwave- safe plastic wrap. Cook on 100% power (high) for 6 to 7 minutes or until turkey is tender and no longer pink, rearranging once.

Cover to keep war.

For sauce, in a 4 cup measure stir together sugar, vinegar and cornstarch.

Stir in tomato, zucchini, green onions and chili peppers. Cook, uncovered on high for 5 to 7 minutes or until mixture is thickened and bubbly, stirring after every minute. Cook on high 1 minute more. Stir over turkey.

Serve with hot cooked rice.

Makes 4 servings
Each serving provides = 1 protein, 1 vegetable, 1 starch, 1 fat

Enjoy!

MICROWAVE MAIN DISH
CITRUS CHICKEN OR TURKEY

Ingredients

12 to 16oz of skinless chicken or turkey breast
½ tsp finely shredded lemon or lime peel
1 tbsp. honey
1 tbsp. soy sauce
1/3 cup orange juice
2 tsp cornstarch
2 medium oranges, peeled and sectioned

Directions:

Rinse chicken; pat dry. Arrange chicken in an 8+8+2- inch baking dish, tucking under thin portions of chicken to make an even thickness.

In a mixing bowl combine lemon or lime juice, honey and soy sauce.

Pour over chicken. Cover with vented microwave-safe plastic wrap.

Cook on 100% power (high) for 4 to 6 minutes or until chicken is tender or no longer pink, rearranging and turning chicken over after 3 minutes.

Remove chicken from dish, reserving juices in dish. Cover chicken to keep warm.

For sauce: combine orange juice and cornstarch; stir into reserved juices.

Cook, uncovered, on high for 2 to 3 minutes or until thickened and bubbly, stirring after every minute until slightly thickened then every 30 seconds. Stir in orange sections. Cook uncovered, on high for 30 to 60 seconds more, or until heated through; spoon over chicken.

Makes 4 servings
Each serving provides = 1 protein, ½ fruit, 1 fat

Enjoy!

CHICKEN KABOBS WITH GINGER LEMON MARINADE

This tart yet sweet marinade complements veal and firm white fish too. For a change try a combination of red or yellow pepper instead of the green pepper. Enjoy!

Ingredients

8oz boneless skinless chicken breasts; cut into 2-inch cubes
16 squares sweet green pepper
16 pineapple chunk (fresh or canned)
16 cherry tomatoes

Ginger lemon marinade
3 tbsp. lemon juice
2 tbsp. water
1 tbsp. vegetable oil
2 tsp sesame oil
1 ½ tsp red wine vinegar
4 tsp brown sugar
1 tsp minced gingerroot (or ¼ tsp ground)
½ tsp ground coriander
½ tsp ground fennel seeds (optional)

Ginger lemon marinade: in a small bowl, combine lemon juice, water, vegetable oil, sesame oil, vinegar, brown sugar, ginger, coriander and fennel seeds (if using); mix well. Add chicken and mix well; marinate for 20 minutes.

Alternately thread chicken cubes, green pepper, pineapple and tomatoes onto 4 long or 8 short barbecue skewers. Barbecue for 15 to 20 minutes or just until chicken is no longer pink inside, brushing often with marinade and rotating every 5 minutes.

Makes 4 servings
Each serving provides = 1 protein, 2 vegetables, 1 fat

Enjoy!

CHICKEN WITH MUSTARD SEED SAUCE

Ingredients

4 chicken fillets, skinless
½ cup tomato sauce
1 tsp tabasco sauce
1tbsp. Worcestershire sauce
2 tbsp. seeded mustard
1 tbsp. brown vinegar
1 clove garlic crushed

Preheat oven temperature: 350%F

Arrange chicken in casserole

Combine tomato sauce, tabasco sauce, mustard, Worcestershire sauce, vinegar and garlic.

Pour over chicken.

Cover and bake for 45 minutes.

Serve with cooked rice and vegetables or salad.

Makes 4 servings
Each serving provides = 1 protein, ¼ vegetable

Enjoy!

BEEF CURRY:
(YOU CAN ALSO USE CHICKEN OR TURKEY BREAST).

Ingredients

1 lb lean beef
Ground black pepper
2 tsp oil (optional)
1 large onion peeled and chopped
2 potatoes scrubbed and chopped
½ cup skinned and chopped pumpkin
½ cup peeled and chopped sweet potato
2 medium zucchini cut into chunks
1 tsp dried coriander
1 tsp dried cumin
½ tsp dried cardamom
2 tsp mustard seeds
½ to 1 tsp dried ground chilies
2 tsp finely chopped or minced garlic
2 tsp finely chopped or minced fresh ginger
1 cup water
Pinch of sea salt, to taste (optional)

Directions: preheat oven to 400%F.

Trim any fat from meat. Cut into 1-inch cubes and sprinkle with pepper.

In a frying pan, fry (or sauté in 2 tsp of hot oil) until browned on all sides. Set aside in bowl.

In the same frying pan sauté the vegetables and set aside with the meat.

Now add to the frying pan the dry spices and cook for 3-4 minutes over medium heat to release the fragrance, and then add the ginger and garlic.

Add water and stir the pan juices well.

Return meat and vegetables to pan, add salt if desired, and stir to combine the flavors.

Spoon into casserole, cover and cook in the oven for approximately 1 to 2 hours until meat is tender.

To store: cover and refrigerate for up to 4 days

Makes 4-5 servings

Each serving provides = 1 protein, ½ vegetables, 1 starch, ½ fat

Enjoy!

UNROLLED CABBAGE ROLLS

Ingredients

¾ cup chopped onions
1 clove garlic, minced
1 ½ cups chicken stock
¾ cup uncooked ling grain white rice
1 medium head cabbage (about 3-4 pounds)
1 ½ pound lean ground turkey (skinless)
1 egg
¼ cup chopped fresh parsley
1 tsp marjoram
½ tsp each sea salt and black pepper
2 cans (10 ounces each) tomato soup

Directions:

Spray a medium saucepan with non-stick spray. Add onions and garlic. Cook over medium heat for 2 minutes, stirring often.

Add broth and rice. Bring to a boil. Reduce heat to medium – low.

Cover and cook for 20 to 25 minutes, until rice is tender and liquid has been absorbed. Stir occasionally.

Meanwhile, bring a large pot of water to a boil. Cut cabbage into 8 wedges. Boil cabbage wedges for 5 minutes. Drain. Remove tough inner pieces. Separate individual leaves and set aside.

Combine cooked rice with turkey, egg, parsley, marjoram, salt and pepper.

Mix well (using your hands works best).

Spray a 13+9 – inch baking pan with non-stick spray. Line bottom with ½ the cabbage leaves. Spread rice/turkey mixture evenly over cabbage. Top with remaining cabbage leaves. Empty both cans of soup into a medium bowl. Add a can of water and mix well.

Pour soup evenly over cabbage. Cover and bake for 1 hour at 350%F. reduce heat to 325%F. and cook another 45 minutes. Let cool for 5 minutes before serving.

Makes 8 servings
Each serving provides = 1 protein, 1 vegetable, 1 starch, 1 fat

Enjoy!

GRILLED SALMON WITH ORANGE GLAZE

Total prep & cooking time: 15 minutes

Ingredients

½ cup orange marmalade
2 tsp grated fresh ginger root
1 garlic clove, crushed
3 tbsp. white rice vinegar (or other vinegar)
1 pound boneless, skinless salmon fillet cut in four pieces
6 thinly sliced scallions with some green (optional)
¼ cup toasted sesame seeds (optional)
Directions;

Combine marmalade, oil, soy sauce, ginger, garlic and vinegar
Heat grill: brush orange glaze on each side of salmon and grill
About 5 minutes on each side. Top with scallions and sesame seeds and serve.

Makes 4 servings
Each serving provides = 1 protein, ½ fat

Enjoy!

MICROWAVE MAIN DISH
CURRIED CHICKEN OR TURKEY CASSEROLE

Ingredients

1-8oz can pineapple chunks (juice pack)
3 cups loose-pack frozen cauliflower, broccoli and carrots
¼ cup water
8oz boned skinless chicken or turkey breast cut into bite size strips
8oz plain yogurt
2 tbsp. all-purpose flour
2 to 3 tsp curry powder
½ tsp sea salt

Drain pineapple, reserving juice; set aside

In a 2- quart casserole combine frozen vegetables and water. Cook, covered, on 100% power (high) for 4 to 6 minutes or until vegetables are nearly thawed, stirring once. Drain.

Stir in chicken and reserved pineapple juice. Cook uncovered, on high for 5 to 8 minutes or until chicken is no longer pink, stirring once.

Meanwhile, for sauce, stir together yogurt, flour, curry powder and salt; stir into casserole. Cook, uncovered on high for 4 to 7 minutes or until sauce is thickened and bubbly, stirring after every minute. Stir in pineapple chunks.

Cook, uncovered, on high for 30 seconds or till heated through.

Makes 4 servings
Each serving provides = 1 protein, 1 ½ vegetables, ½ fat

Enjoy!

CHILLI CON CARNE

Ingredients

1 lb ground chicken or turkey
1cup chopped onion
1 cup finely chopped celery
½ cup finely chopped green bell pepper
16oz can tomatoes, cut up with liquid
1 ¼ tsp sea salt
2 cloves garlic, minced
½ tsp dried oregano
1 tbsp. chilli powder (more if desired)
16oz can kidney beans, with liquid
1 cup water

Directions:

Sauté chicken or turkey in a medium sized non-stick pot: until no pink remains.

Drain in colander to remove fat; return to pot. Add onion, celery and green pepper; mix well. Cover and cook over medium heat 2-3 minutes. Bring to a boil; cover and reduce heat to low, simmer gently 25 minutes, stirring occasionally.

Makes 6 servings = 1 cup
Each serving provides = 1 protein, 1 starch, 1 vegetable

Enjoy!

COOKING TIP

Ground turkey or chicken bought from supermarket often contains ground skin which can increase fat content substantially. For the leanest ground turkey or chicken, grind it yourself. Remove all visible fat before grinding. If you don't have a meat grinder, cut the turkey or chicken into cubes and finely chop in a food processor. Or better yet, ask the butcher to grind the skinless turkey or chicken breast for you.

GRILLED PORK CHOPS

Ingredients

6 pork chops, trimmed of fat 4 to 5oz each
1 cup V8 juice
3 cloves garlic, minced
2 tbsp. brown sugar
1 ½ tbsp. Worcestershire sauce
1 ½ tsp each chili powder and ground cumin
¾ tsp dried oregano
½ tsp black pepper

Directions:

Arrange pork chops in a single layer in a shallow pan
Combine remaining ingredients and pour over pork chops
Turn pork chops to coat both sides with marinade
Cover and marinate in refrigerator for at least 8 hours or overnight
Preheat grill. Cook pork chops over hot coals for 6 to 7 minutes on each side, basting with any leftover marinade.
Serve with rice and vegetables

Makes 6 servings
Each serving provides = 1 protein, 1 fat

Enjoy!

When you have reached your goal weight and have balanced out over a week it is time to start to stabilize your body by introducing foods you have not eaten while you were losing weight. This is where you will learn that 85 to 90 percent of what we eat does not do us any harm; it's the repetitive act that hangs around.

What I want you to do is write out a list of what you would like to try while in stabilization as it can take four to six weeks to stabilize your body; and be able to maintain goal weight for the rest of your life.

What I suggest is you try one thing at a time giving your body 48 hours to go back to goal weight. So for example (you try Pizza) on Friday and let's say you weigh yourself on Saturday and you are up 1 or 2 lbs don't worry pizza is a prime example of high fats high sodium (salt) and remember it takes 48 hours to break that down if however it is still in your system meaning you are still holding after 48 hours it is reacting like a foreign body in your body; meaning it's got no nutritional value; just fats and bad ones at that. So if it is something you like at least when you do eat it you will know how long it takes to get rid of it.

Stabilizing your body is a lot of fun it actually is my favourite part of the program it is where you learn a lot about yourself and the foods you were eating. Hopefully while working hard losing your weight your food choices have changed. But you still need to stabilize to find out what the other foods do to your body.

Try a different food every three days giving your body time to adapt. This is where you learn about the foods you used to eat what ones will enhance your body meaning they leave after 24 hours and what ones don't. The ones that hang around you should be aware of when you are going to eat so as you do not eat the left overs the next day; that would be the repetitive act, and poor eating. Remember old habits die hard. So don't fall back. Try something and then pull back on track with your program so as you stay on track with the new eating patterns you have been following while you were losing weight. The more you do this the easier it will be.

STABILIZATION & MAINTAINANCE

Behaviourial Guidance Material

Part 1

Low fat on the run: = Eating on the run is a way of life for almost everyone. Unfortunately, it is also one of the best ways to undermine a proper diet. This is because it is predicted on grab and go nutrition that all too often means; fast food that is high in fat and calories. When time is tight and hunger strikes, the only alternative for many of us is to seek out the nearest deli, pizzeria or fast food shop. Once In we usually take a perfunctory look around and then make a quick grab for a couple of pepperoni slices perhaps a bacon cheese burger and fries or a tuna salad on rye with chips. There might even be one last high fat grab as we spy that particularly attractive chocolate chip cookie or apple fruit square.

Balance, moderation and variety:= Even those who recognise the benefits of reducing fat and maintaining a balanced diet often see their best laid plans fall prey to the pitfalls of the salad bar or the misleading labels on low- fat muffins, sandwiches and snacks.

Fortunately, there is hope for eliminating fat even for the busiest among us and it doesn't mean rearranging your lifestyle or spending hours at home preparing mobile low fat meals. It also doesn't mean becoming a lifetime member of the nearest "sprouts are people too" restaurant. What it does require, however, is a greater understanding of your food choices and the ability to alter your approach to eating. "It really comes down to balance, moderation and variety".

It's not only altering what you eat, but how you eat it. For example, it is important to control portion size no matter what you are eating. This can be pretty difficult when the size of your meal is determined by someone on the other side of a counter, especially if it is a deli given to incredible generosity. What is the option? Either ask for a smaller portion, share what you're getting or try to eat half of what you buy.

Low Fat On The Run

Part 2

Portion control: = Luckily, limiting fat doesn't mean giving up all of your high fat favourites. But it does mean being aware of portions fat content and making some accommodations, for example, if you want that piece of cake or double crust pie go ahead, but stop at one piece, skip the ice cream or whipped cream topping. Offset the impact of having that pie by eating fresh fruit at your next meal. "Take it one step at a time". If you try to do it all at once, you can get overwhelmed and frustrated and give up too early.

Breakfast : = Take a piece of fresh fruit and some yogurt with you as you leave the house; even if you don't have a stash at home, these are usually available at the nearest deli or food store.

Stay away from croissants, which are high in fat, if you feel like having some bread. Go instead for a bagel or English muffin, but remember to consider portions, especially when buying bagels. They keep getting bigger every day, so now your standard bagel is really a jumbo bagel, which is the equivalent of four to six slices of bread. Remember to look before you leap.

Avoid high fat spreads: = cream cheese and butter are particularly detrimental choices. To make matters worse, delis tend to spread them on by the pound. Either ask for a thin smear, or better yet keep some at your office so you can control the amount. Fruit spreads like apple butter are an even better choice.

Beware of the ever popular muffin: = muffins are high in fat and like bagels getting bigger all the time. So if you want a muffin, reach for the smaller one and don't slather it with butter. Watch out for the "low fat muffins" they can also create problems because often there is no way of telling exactly how much fat they hold, despite their claims many are still relatively high in fat and loaded with calories.

Substitute Canadian bacon for American bacon: = if you are going out for traditional breakfast of bacon and eggs. It is much lower in fat. And skip the home fries and the butter on your toast. Go for pancakes instead of French toast or waffles. French toast has more than twice the fat of pancakes, and waffles have three to four times the amount. Use half in half or whole milk in your coffee instead of cream. Over time the fat savings can add up.

Low Fat On The Run

Part 3

Lunch = Shun mayonnaise-based sandwiches- such as, tuna, chicken, turkey, shrimp and crab salad. They are arch-enemies for anyone cutting down on fat.

Instead fill sandwiches with lean meat such as turkey, chicken, (or roast beef) some cuts of pork and ham and hold the mayo. Avoid adding cheese to your meat sandwiches. Use lettuce tomatoes and onions instead. Try mustard, horseradish or a chutney as a substitute for mayonnaise.

Beware of salad bars = they present an unexpected challenge because they are usually stocked with vast varieties of high fat foods. Go for vegetables, fresh fruit, plain tuna, crab meat or shrimp. Skip noodle dishes in oil or sauces, tuna or chicken salads hard boiled eggs olives avocados grated cheese bacon bits ham chunks coleslaw and marinated vegetables. Also pass on the hot dishes like meat loaf fried chicken and macaroni and cheese.

Eliminate salad bar dressings = they are also high in fat; so for Italian, ranch or yogurt. They usually have about one fifth to one eighth the amount of fat of their full fat counterparts. Order pizza with fresh vegetable topping instead of pepperoni, sausage or meat balls, which can easily double a slice's content.

Order your burgers plain; and pass up on the French fries. Consider that a bacon cheeseburger weighs in at about 27 grams of fat while a cheese burger has 14 grams and a plain hamburger has 12 grams. If you toss in fries, you're adding another 12 gram. By the way a hot dog has 15 gram of fat!

Try rotisserie chicken, but reduce the fat content further by removing the skin. On the other hand, the side dishes offered by the rotisserie emporiums, like creamed spinach, mashed potatoes and macaroni and cheese are high in fat.

Stay away from the heavily fried food Chinese restaurants, shun lo-mien, fried rice or egg rolls, spareribs are also pretty fatty. On the other hand soups, chopsuey, and stir fry dishes are relatively low fat.

I'm really not trying to spoil your day. Just letting you know so you can decide.

LOW FAT ON THE RUN

Part 3 page 2

Snacks: = go for fresh carrots or celery especially if you're tense and want to work of some anxiety by crunching away. Many delis now carry prepared snacks.

Choose relatively low-fat snack foods, such as fresh fruit, spiced applesauce, 2% yogurt, or frozen fruit bars.

If you're in need of something that seems a bit more decadent, go for pretzels-both hard and soft or baked tortilla chips and salsa. If cake is a must, opt for a small slice of angel food cake. Avoid corn or potato chips, ice cream, doughnuts and milkshakes. And oh yes, don't let that thin piece of pound cake deceive you- it is extremely high in fat.

Dinner = Dinner on the run usually means a restaurant where it is often difficult to assess the fat content of various dishes. Even descriptions of low fat items on the menu don't always help, unless they are providing specific information. Skip anything with a cream cheese or sauce because it's going to be relatively high in fat. Beware of words on a menu, like pan fried, buttery, sautéed, with gravy, hollandaise sauce or au gratin. They signal that a dish may be high in fat.

Stick with menu items that are – grilled, steamed, poached, broiled, braised or blackened. They stand a better chance of being lower in fat.

Limit the bread and butter you eat before your meal arrives.

Go for low fat appetizers – like soup, shrimp cocktail, or salad without dressing.

Be wary of French onion soup – if it's covered with cheese a simple cup could have 100 calories and 8 grams of fat.

Always ask for salad dressing or sauces on the side. When you do you are in control of how much you use. Control is what it's all about.

Low fat on the run = choose fresh fruit with perhaps a very small dollop of whipped cream on the side once in a while for desert.

Avoid bake goods with frosting. Double cream or double crusts; cheesecake as you may guess is loaded with fat.

Trick your taste buds = for buttery tasting popcorn without the fat or calories, sprinkle popped kernels with water.

Know the scoop = before eating soup, throw in a few ice cubes to make the fat rise or refrigerate overnight so it hardens at the top. Then skim of the fatty layer.

Pasta is a complex carbohydrate that supplies six of the eight essential amino acids. Although it's loaded with B vitamins and iron, it's not loaded with fat- one cup of cooked pasta has only 1 gram of fat and 210 calories. But like a salad or baked potato, inherently low – fat pasta can be corrupted by what you put on it; which can add significant fat content to pasta dishes. Alfredo sauces are typically made with whipping cream, which has 5 grams of fat per tablespoon. Look for tomato based sauces or ones that specifically indicate that they are lower in fat. Being choosy about pasta sauces and how they are prepared is a very simple way to slice away unnecessary fat- a small investment that pays big health dividends.

You've been a nutritional saint for a while now, eating sensible, low fat foods and exercising four or five times a week. You feel and look great. Now the big challenge you're faced with your first real test of character, your first confrontation with a high fat, high calorie, rip roaring, gut busting pig out – situation – eating at a restaurant! Your friend orders the Godzilla burger with fries and gravy. The other orders the prime rib special. You salivate, thinking "ah what the heck" what's a few extra calories, anyway, just remember that one "ah what the heck" restaurant meal can amount to over 1500 calories that'll wind up around middle; and after throwing caution to the wind even once, it's easy to talk yourself into doing it again and again.

GO FOR QUALITY & QUANTITY!

If you choose to eat a minuscule OZ of polish sausage'
You're choosing a remarkable 32 grams of fat.
The equivalent of eating 128 cups of popcorn;

If you choose to eat a paltry 1oz of Colby cheese,
You'll be choosing a whopping 9 grams of fat.
The equivalent of eating 30 bowls of Kellogg's corn flakes, with milk.
Which would fill you up more?

If you choose to eat 1 burger king double whopper,
You'll be choosing a whopping 53 grams of fat.
The equivalent of eating 5,300 grapes;
Which would fill you up more?

If you choose to eat one meagre cinnamon bun with icing,
You'll be choosing a tremendous 34 grams of fat.
The equivalent of eating 22 slices of raisin bread;
Which would fill you up more?

You'd have to oink out on 37 cups of fresh pineapple,
To consume the 26 grams of fat;
Found in a mere ½ cup peanut butter chocolate ice cream.
Which would fill you up more?

If you choose to eat a measly 1 tablespoon of mayonnaise,
You'll be choosing a whopping 11 grams of fat;
The equivalent of eating 157 cups of raspberries;
Which would fill you up more?

You'd have to oink out on 15 cans of water packed tuna,
To consume the 12 grams of fat;
Found in a paltry 3 slices of bacon;
Which would fill you up more?
You'd have to oink out on 500 steamed shrimp,
To consume the 25 grams of fat;
Found in 1 sausage egg Mcmuffin;
Which would fill you up more?

If you choose to eat a minuscule 1oz of pepperoni,
You'll be choosing a remarkable 12 grams of fat;
The equivalent of eating 60 sweet peppers;
Which would fill you up more?

You'd have to oink out on 150 cups of honeydew melon,
To consume the 30 grams of fat, found in a mere 2 pieces
Off fresh coconut (2"+2"+1/2)
Which would fill you up more?

If you choose to eat a feeble 2 slices of Bologna,
You'll be choosing a mammoth 16 grams of fat;
The equivalent of eating 16 cups of rigatoni;
Which would fill you up more?

If you choose to nibble on 1 honey-dipped cruller,
You'll be choosing a walloping 11 grams of fat.
The equivalent of eating 11 slices of whole wheat toast;
Which would fill you up more?

If you choose to eat a trifling ½ cup of dry roasted pistachios,
You'll be choosing an unbelievable 34 grams of fat.
The equivalent of eating 34 cobs of corn;
Which would fill you up more?

You'd have to oink out on 23 whole pitas,
To consume the 16 grams of fat found in ½ cup French onion chip dip.
Which would fill you up more?

If you choose to eat 1 scoop of French vanilla ice cream,
You're choosing 18 grams of fat.
The equivalent of eating 450 Carmel rice cakes: Which would fill you up more?
If you choose to eat a scrawny 1 tablespoon of margarine,
You'll be choosing a surprising 11 grams of fat.
The equivalent of eating 12 cups of boiled lobster;
Which would fill you up more?

You'd have to oink out on 200 pretzel twists,
To consume the 20 grams of fat, found in 1 hot dog.
Which would fill you up more?

You'd have to oink out on 37 kiwi fruit,
To consume the 13 grams of fat found in.
1 package of Reese's peanut butter cups;
Which would fill you up more?

If you choose to eat 1 measly apple turnover,
You'll be choosing 17 grams of fat.
The equivalent of eating 17 cups of spaghetti;
Which would fill you up more?

If you choose to eat one meager restaurant-style egg roll,
You'll be choosing a total 6 grams of fat.
The equivalent of eating 60 fresh peaches;
Which would fill you up more?

If you choose to eat a measly ½ cup of regular trail mix,
You'll be choosing an incredible 22 grams of fat.
The equivalent of eating 56 bowls of Kellogg's rice krispies with milk;
Which would fill you up more?

You'd have to oink out on 110 oranges,
To consume the 20 grams of fat; found in 1 hotdog.
Which would fill you up more?

If you choose to eat a paltry ½ cup of sunflower seeds,
You'll be choosing a whopping 35 grams of fat.
The equivalent of eating 2 entire loaves of multigrain bread;
Which would fill you up more?

You'd have to oink out on 146 cups of cream of wheat,
To consume the 44 grams of fat found in a mere;
½ cup of whipping cream.
Which would fill you up more?

If you choose to eat 1 medium order of fries,
You'll be choosing a gut busting 16 grams of fat.
The equivalent of eating 80 cups of yams;
Which would fill you up more?

You'd have to oink out on 100 baked potatoes,
To consume the 10 grams of fat found in a measly,
1 ounce of potato chips (an average handful);
Which would fill you up more?

If you choose to eat a measly 2 gourmet-style semi-sweet
Chocolate chip cookies, you'll be choosing a humungous 21 grams of fat.
The equivalent of eating 35 cups of wild rice;
Which would fill you up more?

You'd have to oink out on 17 bananas
To consume the 17 grams of fat, found in 1 cup of eggnog.
Which would fill you up more?

You'd have to oink out on 31 cups of fresh strawberries,
To consume the 19 grams of fat found in;
1 plain croissant;
Which would fill you up more?

Remember to go for quality as well as quantity!

Children and weight gain and weight loss like I have said earlier in this book children see; children do. They mimic their parents or care givers so if you or a care giver has an eating problem meaning feed yourself one day and starve the next the possibility of your child following in your footsteps is very possible, let's change that. The program I have designed for 12 year olds to 16 years has worked for thousands of children and teenagers. I always say small changes work best. Changing a few of our items in our grocery cart

Stage three of program

Diet plan for youth 12to 16 years old = medium to large frame

Entrees or protein = 2 serving daily
Vegetables = 4 servings daily
Fruit = 4 servings daily
Starches = 5 servings daily
Fats = 2 servings daily
Milk = 8oz daily
½ cup un-popped popcorn morning, afternoon or evening use it whenever you need it.

Keep track of foods eaten on your food diary for yourself: that way you will know what you are eating daily so as not to over eat or under eat; weigh and measure foods; you need to develop the eye for serving size. I like to think we are ok at home; you can't bring the scales to a restaurant or someone' home when you go out. So being able to look at your plate without saying anything to see if there is too much of one thing and not enough of another, lets you know what you are going to leave on your plate, or what you can have more off.

Don't worry it will get easier and less confusing as the weeks pass; you will have more confidence in yourself; and honestly that is the best feeling in the world.

I personally do not put children under the age of 12 on a diet or food plan.

The best way to help; your child or children is to change what you buy at the grocery store.

Honestly you will find that going grocery shopping, picking the foods you and your family will enjoy, knowing in your heart that you are doing something really good for your family.

Take your time shopping, stop picking up food that is ready to eat in five minutes or less; start to look before you put it in the shopping cart, instead of going for chips and dips cookies ETC; pick up some vegetables, fruit and yogurt.

Make your own dips chop it up and leave in the fridge make some jello or puddings that they can have when they get home if you leave it ready on the counter or in the fridge believe me they will eat it.

Eating the junk is a habit for them; it's what's there and easy for them. The great thing with children is that they can break old patterns easily and they don't even realise that they are doing it.

You don't have to say were making changes no more junk because that makes them feel like they did something wrong. Just do it, say nothing, if you want cookies make them yourself; at least you will know what is in them.

Taking the little bit of time cooking it and knowing what you are putting on the table is good and nutritious. You will save money and have a healthier family. Start to make going out to eat something special, that you all do together, or put what you save away and take a nice family holiday.

You have to start somewhere.

Sure you will find that something's you cook don't turn out the way you wanted or you could say that's absolutely disgusting; I have said it myself and I'm a pretty good cook. That's ok next time it will be better, don't give up remember why you are doing this. Just take a big deep breath at those times and start all over again, be able to laugh at you self; when it turns out perfect you will be quite proud of yourself. You will just get better and better.

OBESITY is worldwide and fast food has a lot to do with it; when you bring home dinner, it's usually fast food, and usually eaten alone. Either in the bedroom or games room, why because you're tired: you worked all day and they are watching TV or on the computer. We need to get involved most habits that form in children start at school where they get a real education and you know what I mean. If they are not talking to you and learning from you, then they are getting it elsewhere.

CHILDREN AND FOOD

I'm sure you have heard the old saying breakfast is the most important meal of the day. Why you may say, 1. It wakens the body and brain up for the day.

2. Wakens up foods eaten the night before (Starts body up).3 energy.

Three important facts; are your children eating a nutritious breakfast? I don't think so.

There are a lot of reasons for my thinking this. Half the time; we are not home for breakfast we are already at work or on the way. More children are seeing themselves off to school, so what are they eating. I would say 50% are eating something the other 50% nothing. They are going to school tired, cold and hungry. It's no wonder they are not paying attention in class they don't have the fuel in them to charge their body.

We need to change this. Children eating pop tarts, pizza pockets, chocolate, donuts, bagels, etc. yes you got it junk food no nutritional value; all that will do overtime is make more obese children which causes problems for them as they go through school. This really is a serious problem. Having a weight problem as an adult is hard enough. Having one as a child is disastrous for many different reasons; first and foremost is the child's health.

So moms and dads what are you going to do?

Now I understand you can't do what you don't know read on I'm going to help you. We need to start with ourselves, because if we can fix ourselves we can do anything right!

If as mothers and fathers, let's not leave them out; they are a big factor here too.

If we really don't know what we are doing then it's better to start at the beginning. I think so anyway.

If as a child you can think, what did I have for breakfast and smile to yourself, then you probably had someone in your life that when you got up in the morning had breakfast on the table ready for you, porridge if it was cold outside; fruit and cereal, bacon and egg or bread and jam. If not and you remember getting up and nothing was on the table, you probably had pop tarts or nothing at all, you would have gone to school hungry, I am sorry for that. We can't go back; so let's step forward because I can help you. Remember you can't do what you don't know.

When we are born we come into the world perfect, we depend on our parents to keep us safe we look to them for everything they are our teachers. Remember that children can only do what they see and they take the good and the bad with them.

If you were born fifty or sixty years ago you also were lucky to have your mom at home the homemaker she was always there got you up in the morning had breakfast ready, made your lunch and when you got home everyone sat down together for dinner. Today things are quite different and that's just life; times have changed so much it takes two working now to bring up a family.

We only have a short time to teach our children and keep them on the right track. So once again I will say this breakfast is the most important meal of the day. Tomorrow get up half an hour earlier and make something for you and your children, have it on the table, you will notice the difference right away.

HOW TO HELP YOUR CHILDREN TO MAINTAIN A HEALTHY WEIGHT

There is no magic bullet when it comes to weight loss for children. The best approach is a general approach which incorporates the following.

Encourage your child to make changes to their general lifestyle.

Encourage him or her to become more physically active.

Make it easy for him or her to eat healthy.

Set a good example for him or her, yourself.

Encourage your child to make changes to their general lifestyle.

Less television, less computer,

Several studies have found a strong link between obesity and time watching TV.

This isn't surprising.

We burn fewer calories watching television than we do sitting still.

TV commercials urge viewers to eat.

The average child sees 10,000 TV commercials a year. Approx. 9,500 of these are for one of four types of food: fast food, soft drinks, sugar coated cereals and candy.

Too much TV is bound to prevent kids from developing the skills and love of sports that make physical activity so enjoyable.

Playing computer games may be worse than simply watching TV. Not only can they become addictive, but they can be played all day and night.

LESS TELEVISION FOR PARENTS TOO:

We parents rely on TV to amuse our children. Then we get upset when our kids get fat. The moral; we have to take a greater interest in our children, and their activities. This doesn't mean we have to entertain our children from morning till night. But we have to get involved.

We should encourage our older children to read, do something creative or participate in school or community sports and activities.

We should set aside more time to play with our younger children.

We should set an example by talking to our children about different things, in the hope that we can interest and inspire them to undertake new activities and projects.

ENCOURAGE YOUR CHILDREN TO BECOME MORE PHYSICALLY ACTIVE

SUGGESTIONS:

Be active yourself: share your activity with your kids.

Play with them: play football, go cycling, go skating, and go swimming.

Be more active as a family. Take family walks and hikes etc.

Help your children to find activities that they enjoy by showing them different possibilities.

A good trick to encourage them to exercise is to ask them to help you to get fit. Ask them to go for a walk with you, or a swim or a cycle.

MAKE IT EASY FOR THEM TO EAT HEALTHILY:

Be subtle. Even if your children are overweight; don't make a fuss about it. You will only make things worse. The key is to make it easy (and enjoyable) for them to eat properly. You can't force them.

BASIC APPROACH:

Be positive about making changes.

Be encouraging rather than dogmatic.

If there are other children in the family whose weight is normal, don't make an issue of the overweight child having to "go on a diet" while the other kids carry on eating as "normal".

Introduce changes on a "healthy eating" pretext for all the family rather than a "diet" for the overweight child.

Let them know that they are great as they are, and that losing weight is something they can do to improve their life, not something to make other people approve of them.

Talk about the benefits they will get from changing their eating habits. Explain it will make things even better for them e.g. more energy, more confidence, more friends, more clothes and so on.

Talk to them about the changes that they could make. Get them to agree. Don't impose anything.

PRACTICAL SUGGESTIONS:

Provide a range of healthy snacks that the children can grab for themselves- a variety of whole wheat cereals, different breads, fresh fruit, jelly, yogurt, etc.

If they really love junk food, cook your own at home rather than allowing them take outs. Use lean steak to make burgers, serve on a whole wheat bun with lots of salad, and make your own oven chips by cutting potatoes into thick chips, spray with light cooking spray and cook in hot oven.

If they eat at school, find out what choices are available and talk to them about the best choices to make. Be involved that's important. Don't insist they take a packed lunch if this makes them feel uncomfortable. Remember what it was like at school- Kids like to be the same, they don't want to stand out.

Fast foods need not be fattening – buy a pizza base and put your own toppings \chicken/tomato/cottage cheese/peppers/etc.

Mix some 1%milk with whole milk 3% and keep it in a jug; in the fridge.

Make air popped popcorn leave it on the kitchen counter.

If you know your child loves a particular dish which is high in fat, don't cut it out completely. Include it in his/her diet every couple of weeks.

Make a healthy fizzy drink by mixing one-third fruit juice with two-thirds fizzy water.

Get a set of ice-pop molds, fill them with fruit juice and freeze for a delicious cool ice.

Encourage them to use the blender to make their own shakes. Use any soft fruit, banana, peaches, raspberries, strawberries, blend with milk and top with a scoop of frozen yogurt.

For a more sophisticated snack, mix dried fruits with seeds- use sesame seeds or pumpkin seeds. If you see your child eating something fattening, don't make a fuss and don't expect them to be perfect. The occasional bad food isn't going to stop them from losing weight. Remember the most important thing is to teach them long-term, good eating habits.

Don't compare your child in a critical way with anyone else. I'm sure we all remember hearing about so and so being so good at everything, or so clever, or so good looking. Children pick up on these things and what they here is "why aren't you more like so and so.

Constantly talking about weight/dieting, your own or your child's can be very damaging. There are many cases of eating disorders in teenage girls who have grown up in a household where the mother is an obsessive dieter.

Ideally, introduce good eating habits to your child or children as early as possible, but remember it is never too late to start. The wonderful thing about children is that they adapt to new ideas very quickly.

SET A GOOD EXAMPLE FOR YOUR CHILDREN

Most children learn by example, they watch and they copy. One of the most important things you can do to prevent obesity in your child, is to set a good personal example.

Take regular exercise.

Don't sit in front of a TV or computer all day.

Find out about nutrition.
Buy lots of healthy food.
Cook healthy meals.
Explain to your children what makes foods healthy and unhealthy.

Weight problems and obesity in children:

The number of children who are obese or overweight is growing at an alarming rate. Extra pounds put children at risk of serious health problems: For example =type 2 diabetes, heart disease, asthma, bone and joint problems, high cholesterol and liver and gall bladder disease.

Childhood obesity also takes an emotional toll. Overweight children are frequently teased and excluded from team activities, which can lead to low self- esteem, negative body image and depression.

Children who are unhappy with their weight may also be more likely to develop eating disorders and substance abuse problems.

Recognising and dealing with weight problems or obesity in children as early as possible may reduce the risk of them developing these other serious medical conditions as they get older.

Whatever your children's weight, though, let them know that you love them and that all you want to do is help them be healthy and happy.

Understanding how children become obese or overweight in the first place is an important step towards breaking the cycle. Most cases of childhood obesity are caused by eating too much and exercising too little.

Children need enough food to support healthy growth and development. But when they take in more calories than they burn throughout the day, the result is weight gain.

Many factors contribute to this growing imbalance between calories in and calories out. Busy families are cooking less and eating out more: easy access to cheap, high calorie fast food and junk food. Food portions are bigger than they used to be, both in restaurants and at home.

Children are consuming a huge amount of sugar in sweetened drinks and hidden in an array of foods.

Children spend less time actively playing outside, and more time watching TV, playing video games and sitting at the computer.

Many schools are eliminating or cutting back their physical education programs. However, with the right support, encouragement, and positive role modeling, you can help your child reach and maintain a healthy weight. Healthy habits start at home.

The best way to fight or prevent childhood obesity and weight problems is to get the whole family on a healthier track. Making better food choices and becoming more active will benefit everyone, regardless of weight; and with the whole family involved, it will be much easier for your overweight child to make lasting changes.

The most effective way to influence your child is by your own healthy example. If your children see you eating your vegetables, being active, and limiting your TV time, there's a good chance that they will do the same.

These habits will also have the happy side effect of helping you maintain a healthy weight.

Recognize that you have more control than you might think. You can turn of the TV, computer, or video game.

You can choose to walk to the store, especially when you are with your children. You can give your family more vegetables for dinner.

Think about the immediate benefits. If reducing the risk of future heart disease seems abstract, focus on the good things that can happen right now.

You will not feel uncomfortably full if you have a smaller portion or skip desert.

Going hiking with your teenager might lead to a wonderful talk that neither of you anticipated. A fruit salad tastes great and looks beautiful. Dancing or playing with your children is lots of fun and can give you a great workout. Take a walk after dinner a couple nights a week instead of turning on the TV, and instead of chocolate cake with frosting, enjoy sliced strawberries over angel food cake.

Making healthier food choices for your children

Serve and encourage consumption of a wide variety of fruits and vegetables. This should include red (beets, and tomatoes) orange (carrots and squash) yellow (potatoes and banana) green (lettuce and broccoli).

Look for hidden sugar. Reducing the amount of candy and deserts you and your children eat is only part of the battle since sugar is also hidden in foods as diverse as bread, canned soups and vegetables, pasta sauce, margarine, instant mashed potatoes, frozen dinners, fast food and ketchup.

Your body gets all it needs from sugar naturally occurring in food so anything added amounts to nothing but empty calories.

Check labels and opt for low sugar products and use fresh or frozen ingredients instead of canned goods.

Schedule regular meal times: the majority of children like routine. If your child knows they will only get food at certain times, they will be more likely to eat what they get when they get it.

Limit eating out: if you must eat out, avoid fast food if you can and make the healthy choices you are trying to make at home.

Not all fats contribute to weight gain; so instead of trying to cut out fat from your child's diet, focus on replacing unhealthy fats with healthy fats.

French fries and other fried foods may contain artificial trans- fats that are dangerous to your child's health, fast food, packaged food, baked goods, sweets and anything fried in vegetable oil often contain trans-fat, even if the packaging claims that it is "trans- fat-free."

Try to eliminate or cut back on; commercially baked goods (cookies, crackers, cakes, muffins, pie crusts, pizza dough and bread like hamburger buns). Packaged snack foods (microwave popcorn, chips, candy). Solid fats (stick margarine, vegetable shortening). Fried foods: (French fries fried chicken, chicken nuggets, breaded fish and hard taco shells). Pre –mix products cake mix and pancake mix) and anything with "partially hydrogenated "oil listed in the ingredients.

Add more healthy fats: eat foods rich in monounsaturated and polyunsaturated fat is an important part of a healthy diet and can help a child control blood sugar and avoid diabetes. These "good" fats include: Avocados, olives, olive oil, and nuts such as almonds, peanuts, macadamia nuts, pecans, hazelnuts, cashews and walnuts. Fatty fish: such as; salmon, tuna, mackerel, herring, trout, sardines or sablefish. Non –GMO sources of soy and tofu. Brussels sprouts, kale and spinach, Sunflower, sesame, pumpkin seeds and flaxseed.

When cooking for you and your child, choose oils carefully. Cold-pressed oils such as extra virgin oil, sesame oil, and peanut oil are rich in healthy fats. The same may not be true of modern processed oils such as soybean oil, sunflower oil, corn oil, canola oil, cottonseed oil, safflower oil and vegetable oil. These oils are industrially manufactured- usually from genetically modified crops in the US - using high heat and toxic solvents to extract the oil from the seeds. Stick to cold –pressed oils or using butter for cooking and baking.

Not all saturated fat is the same. The saturated fat in whole milk, coconut oil or salmon is different to the saturated fat found in pizza, French fries, and processed meat such as, (ham, sausage, hot dogs, salami, and other cold cuts) which have been linked to heart disease and cancer.

Despite the saturated fat content, children who eat whole –milk dairy products tend to have less body fat and lower levels of obesity that those who eat skim or non –fat dairy. This may be because the saturated fat in whole milk dairy makes children feel fuller, faster, and keeps them feeling satisfied for longer, helping them to eat less. Adding a small amount of butter or olive oil to vegetables will not only improve the taste but can be far more satisfying to children.

Help your child to make healthier choices, focus on the source of saturated fats consumed. A glass of whole milk or natural cheese rather than a hot dog, donut or pastry, (for example) grilled chicken, or fish instead of fried chicken, or a 4oz portion of grass-fed beef rather than a burger and fries.

What to avoid. = saturated fat from processed meats, packaged meals, and takeout food.

Don't replace healthy sources of saturated fat with refined carbs of sugary snacks.

Don't eat just red meat (beef, pork, or lamb) vary your children's diet with chicken, eggs, fish, and vegetarian sources of protein.

When you choose to eat red meat, look for "organic" and "grass fed" to avoid antibiotics, growth hormones and GMOs often found in industrially raised meat.

Roast, grill, or slow cook meat and poultry instead of frying.

Allow your children to enjoy full-fat dairy and choose organic milk, cheese, butter and yogurt whenever possible.

Avoid breaded meats and vegetables and deep fried foods.

Your home is where children eat the majority of his or her meals and snacks, so it is vital that your kitchen is stocked with healthy choices and treats.

Don't ban sweets entirely.

While many children's sugar consumption exceeds healthy limits, having a no sweets rule is an invitation for cravings and overindulging when given the chance. Instead limit the amount of cookies, candies, and baked goods your child eats and introduce fruit-based snacks instead.

Soft drinks are loaded with sugar- empty calories- that don't do anything healthy for your child's growing body. Encourage your children to eat a piece of fruit instead children love Satsuma or tangerine oranges; instead of soda offer your child sparkling water with a twist of lime, fresh mint or a splash of fruit juice.

Don't turn snacks into a meal. Limit them to 100 to 150 calories.

Keep a bowl of fruit out for your children to snack on. Offer fruit as a sweet treat. Include frozen juice bars, fruit smoothies, frozen bananas dipped in chocolate and nuts, strawberries and a dollop of whipped cream, fresh fruit added to plain yogurt and sliced apples with peanut butter.

Use sweet –tasting herbs and spices such as mint, cinnamon, allspice or nutmeg to add sweetness to food without the empty calories.

There's a huge disparity in the amount of added sugar between different brands off cereal, even those proclaiming to be whole grain or high in fiber. Some cereals are more than 50% sugar by weight. Try mixing a low sugar, high fiber cereal with you children's favorite sweetened cereal, or add fresh or dried fruit to oatmeal for a natural sweet taste.

Learn what a regular portion size looks like. The portion sizes that you and your family are used to eating may be equal to two or three true servings. Read food labels. Information about serving size and calories can be found on the backs of packaging.

To minimize the temptation of seconds and third helpings, serve food on individual plates, instead of putting serving dishes on the table.

Divide food from large packages into smaller containers. The larger the package, the more people tend to eat without realizing it limit daily screen time. The more time your children spend watching TV, playing video games or using computers or mobile devices; the less time they'll spend on active pastimes. Studies show a link between screen time and obesity, so set limits on your children's TV-watching, gaming and web surfing. Experts recommend no more than two hours per day. Stop eating in front of the television, starting now your family does all their eating at the table.

You can make a huge impact on your children's health by being involved with the details of their lives.

Talk to your children; ask them about the school day "everyday" listen to their concerns and take action if there is something they need. Talk to your children's teachers get involved. You don't want to be that parent that here's about their children from the neighbours. You may feel like neither you or your child has time for long chats about the day. This may be the toughest lifestyle change you ever have to make, due to busy schedules, but it can be done.

You don't have to spend all your time having heart to hearts. Playing, reading, cooking or any other activity, when done together, can supply your children with the self-esteem boost he or she may need to make positive changes.

Remember when you make the changes you need to follow through.

Girls weight scale for age and height normal range

Age 2 = weight 22.5 – 32.1 pounds = height 31.5 -36 inches
Age 3 = weight 25.5 – 37.5 pounds = height 34.5-39.5 inches
Age 4 = weight 28.5- 44.1 pounds = height 37-42.5 inches
Age 5 = weight 32.5-52 pounds = height 39.5-45.5 inches
Age 6 = weight 36- 59 pounds = height 42- 48.5 inches
Age 7 = weight 39.5- 68 pounds = height 44.3 – 51.5 inches
Age 8 = weight 44 – 79 pounds = height 46.5 – 54.2 inches
Age 9 = weight 48 – 90 pounds = height 48.5 – 56.5 inches
Age 10 = weight 55 – 104.5 pounds = height 50-58.7 inches
Age 11 = weight 61 – 117 pounds = height 52 – 61 inches
Age 12 = weight 68 – 135 pounds = height 54.5 – 64 inches
Age 13 = weight 75 – 147 pounds = height 57.2 – 66.4 inches
Age 14 = weight 83.5 – 158 pounds= height 58.7 – 67.5 inches
Age 15 = weight 89 – 167 pounds = height 59.5 – 68 inches

Height and weight scale for boys normal range
Age 2 = weight 22.8-33 pounds= height 31.7- 36.3 inches
Age 3 = weight 26.1 – 38.5 pounds = height 35.2-39.8 inches
Age 4 = weight 29 – 44 pounds = height 37.5 – 43.2 inches
Age 5 = weight33 – 52.5 pounds = height 39.8- 45.7 inches
Age 6 = weight 36.5- 59 pounds = height 42.2 – 48.6 inches
Age 7 = weight 40.5 – 68 pounds = height 44.5 – 51.3 inches

Age 8 = weight 45 – 77 pounds = height 46.7- 54.3 inches
Age 9 = weight 49.5 – 88 pounds = height 48.7 – 56.5 inches
Age 10 = weight 56 – 100.5 pounds = height 50.5 = 58.8 inches
Age 11 = weight 60.5 – 114 pounds = height 52 – 61 inches
Age 12 = weight 66.5 – 130 pounds = height 54 – 63.5 inches
Age 13 = weight 74.5 – 144 pounds = height 56.3- 66.6 inches
Age 14 =weight 84 – 159.5 pounds = height 59.1 -69.7 inches
Age 15 = weight 92.5 – 172.5 pounds = height 61.6 – 71.7 inches

These are weight and height weight; the lower are the average, the higher are where you see signs of children being overweight which leads to obesity.

Childhood obesity has more than doubled in children and quadrupled in adolescents in the past thirty years.

Overweight is defined as having excess body weight for a particular height from fat, muscle, bone, water, or a combination of these factors. Obesity is defined as having excess body fat.

Overweight and obesity are the result of "caloric imbalance" too few calories expended for the amount of calories consumed, and are affected by various genetic, behavioral, and environmental factors.

Childhood obesity has both immediate and long – term effects on health and well- being.

Obese youths are more likely to have risk factors for cardiovascular disease, such as high cholesterol or high blood pressure. In a population sample of 5-17 year olds, 70% of obese youth had at least one risk factor for cardiovascular disease.

Obese adolescents are more likely to have pre-diabetes, a condition in which blood glucose levels indicate a high risk for development of diabetes.

Children and adolescents who are obese are at greater risk for bone and joint problems, sleep apnea, and social and psychological problems such as stigmatization and poor self- esteem.

Children and adolescents who are obese are likely to be obese as adults; and are therefore more at risk for adult health problems such as heart disease, type 2 diabetes, stroke, several types of cancer and osteoarthritis. One study showed that children who became obese as early as age 2 were more likely to be obese as adults.

Overweight and obesity are associated with increased risk for many types of cancer, including cancer of the breast, colon, endometrium, esophagus, kidney, pancreas, gall bladder, thyroid, ovary and cervix, and prostrate, as well as multiple myeloma and Hodgkin's lymphoma.

Healthy lifestyle habits, including healthy eating and physical activity, can lower the risk of becoming obese and developing related diseases.

The dietary and physical activity behaviors of children and adolescents are influenced by many sectors of society, including families, communities, schools, childcare settings, medical care providers, government agencies, the media, food and beverage industries and entertainment industries.

Schools play a particularly critical role by establishing a safe and supportive environment with policies and practices that support healthy behaviors.

OBESITY IS A UNIVERSAL PROBLEM AND ONE THAT NEEDS TO BE ADDRESSED SERIOUSELY

There can be no reasonable doubt, concerning the universal role that nutrition plays in the maintenance of a positive state of high grade health and the prevention and treatment of disease. Clinical nutrition is no longer an empirical science. During the past few decades many new facts have been learned to the deprivation and excess of the basic constituents of food and the importance of altered pathways of utilization. A major health hazard in many nations of the world is obesity. It has been estimated that a significant percentage of adult North American population is obese and the problem appears to be getting worse. Being obese increases your risk for developing hypertension, diabetes mellitus, coronary artery disease, high cholesterol, gall bladder disease, obstetrical complications, anesthesia-related complications, degenerative joint disease, physiological disability, certain cancers (colon, rectum, and prostrate in men; uterus, biliary tract, breast, and ovary in women). Thromboembolic disorders, digestive tract disease (gallstones, hiatus hernias), and skin disorders have been well documented. Obesity appears to accelerate the degenerative disease of the aging process. The death rate increases in proportion to the degree of obesity; "morbid obesity" or 100 lbs above the ideal weight is associated with a 6-12 fold increase in mortality rates, although persons with excessive weight of as little as 20 percent or more exhibit increased mortality rates.

Until recently, obesity was considered to be the direct result of a sedentary lifestyle plus chronic ingestion of excess calories. Obese people were blamed for being obese by their friends and families, their employees, their physicians, and even by themselves. Although these factors are undoubtedly the principal cause of obesity in many cases, there is now evidence that many factors may be also involved.

BACKGROUND

Obesity is one of the most prevalent and debilitating chronic diseases in North America. It has been estimated that at least 34 million North Americans are 20% over their ideal body weight. It is well recognized that obesity contributes significantly to both increased individual morbidity and mortality, as well as to increased national health care costs. A recent study found that obesity is a strong independent risk factor for coronary heart disease in middle aged women. Even mild to moderate overweight is associated with a substantial elevation in coronary risk. Weight gain during adulthood is also found to further increase the risk. As much as 70% of the coronary heart disease among women is attributable to the overweight state and is thus potentially preventable. Obesity robs the individual of their productivity and health and the nation of needed health care resources.

Our children to date are on the average heavier and more obese than they were a generation ago. Until recently there has been little therapeutic success in the treatment of obesity. In fact most traditional diet programs have helped only a few individuals to lose a significant amount of weight. To those individuals who do lose some weight almost all of them regain most, if not all of their weight back. Yet we are still infatuated with the mysticism of EASY WEIGHT LOSS and still continue to spend billions of dollars a year on weight loss programs.

Unfortunately most methods of losing weight are hopelessly ineffective and have not adequately addressed the frustrating problem of chronic obesity.

Many of the ever present fad diets that temp frustrated dieters are more harmful psychologically, physiologically and financially than they are effective for achieving weight loss.

The use of surgery for weight loss is associated with significant morbidity and mortality and is only appropriate for the very morbidly obese. Surgical intervention for obesity bypasses the problem instead of solving it.

The same is true for anorectic medications and diet pills which have little record of success, but rather a large record for risks, addiction and bodily harm.

The concept of using the protein sparing modified fast as a therapeutic tool for weight reduction was developed in the early 1970s on reducing the negative nitrogen balance in surgical patients. It was known that when the surgical or critical ill patients sole nutritional support was intravenous glucose, nitrogen losses were significant and could only be minimally reduced (in general this indicated that there was large muscle mass loss). However it was discovered that when amino acids (protein) were added to the intravenous glucose, nitrogen balance could be maintained with results lean muscle preservation.

During fasting or a very low calorie diet the body seeks to minimize its lean tissue (protein) breakdown and nitrogen losses since it is the level of protein and amino acid concentration in lean tissue that is the crucial element for survival, and not fat stores.

During the initial part of fasting the metabolic fuels are quickly changed as signaled by lowering levels of glucose and insulin. As serum insulin levels drop, free fatty acids are released from fat stores and the body begins to change its fuel requirements from glucose to free fatty acids and ketones. In this way, the body's metabolic reorganization results in reduced muscle breakdown.

Falling levels of insulin results in biochemical changes that causes fat which is a form of stored energy, to be now metabolized as a fuel, adipose (fat) tissue, metabolised from storage sites, is utilized as an energy source; either directly as free fatty acids or indirectly as ketone bodies. The body, by shifting its metabolic requirements from carbohydrate to ketone bodies, is thus able to spare its most valuable fuel, protein. Thus ketosis plays an important part in the preservation of lean muscle tissue. Simply put, if the body does not have enough glucose, it makes it from protein (breakdown of muscle tissue) and as the body adapts to the diet, it makes progressively more use of the ketone bodies for energy and gradually less requirements of glucose, which in consequence spares muscle.

Social factors are very important determinants of obesity, particularly among women. For example, obesity is 6 times prevalent among lower-class than among upper-class women. This social relationship is more than co-relationship.

The social class of one's parents is almost as in one's own. Although obesity influences ones social class (lowering it), it cannot have influenced that of one's parents, suggesting that the social class into which a person is born is a powerful determinant of obesity.

Obesity is far more common among lower class than upper- class children.

Economic and other social factors, particularly ethnic and religious, are also closely linked to obesity. The mechanisms appear to be multiple and complex, but differences in lifestyle, and particularly dietary and exercise patterns, probably play a major role.

ENDOCRINE AND METABOLIC FACTORS:

Endocrine and metabolic factors are usually the consequences rather than causes of obesity. An exception is adipose tissue proliferation and hyperadrenocorticism, in which corticosteroid excess leads to increased gluconeogenesis and a correspondingly greater demand of insulin, which stimulates lipogenesis. Even in this condition the proximate cause of weight gain is the same: more calories are consumed than are expended as energy.

PHYSIOLOGIC FACTORS:

The influence of psychological factors on obesity; while many obese persons overeat when emotionally upset, so do many non-obese persons.

For a small number of obese persons psychopathology may be linked to their obesity, especially on young women of upper and middle socioeconomic classes who have been obese since childhood. They may manifest disordered eating patterns and are at high risk for another troublesome syndrome disparagement of the body image. Characteristically, they feel that their bodies are grotesque and loathsome and that others view them with hostility and contempt. This results in self- consciousness and impaired social functioning.

GENETIC FACTORS

Obesity runs in families: 80% of the offspring of 2 obese parents are obese, compared with 40% of 1 obese parent and only 10% of 2 non – obese parents.

At least part of this familial aggregation of obesity is genetically determined.

Twin studies and a recent adoption study have provided strong evidence for the role of genetic factors in human obesity.

PHYSICAL ACTIVITY

Decreased physical activity in affluent societies is often cited as a major factor in the rise of obesity. Caloric requirements are lower with a sedentary life-style, and animal experiments suggest that physical inactivity contributes to obesity also by a paradoxical effect on food intake. Although food intake increases with increasing energy expenditure, food intake may not decrease proportionately when such activity falls below a minimum level; restricting physical activity may actually increase food intake in some people.

MODE OF TREATMENTS

Excluding surgical and dental approaches (gastric bypass, jaw wiring, etc.) and the pharmacological interventions, there are four possible methods of causing weight reduction.

The role of drugs in the treatment of obesity remains controversial. Lack of effectiveness, the presence of significant side effects, and the potential for dependence should discourage usage.

FORMULA DIET

Formula diets for weight reducing come into vogue periodically; America's most celebrated weight loss was announced when a well-known talk show host disclosed to her multi-million television viewers that she had lost 67 lbs in 4 months by consuming a liquid diet. Sadly consumption of these liquid diets has resulted in 100s of deaths. The use of formula diets is simple, since they require no meal planning and no decisions. However, liquid formulas soon become monotonous and are often discarded in favor of another fad. The person will most likely return to previous dietary habits and regain the pounds lost.

CALORIE COUNTING

Formerly, health professionals advocated that obese patients "eat less of everything" on grounds that a weight reduction regimen is more sensible if it is nutritionally balanced and composed of conventional array of foods. Unfortunately, this direct approach, while appearing reasonable, has been effective in only a very small proportion of cases. Why is this so? First of all, calorie counting, which requires careful monitoring of portion sizes, can be difficult and tedious if one consumes a restricted variety of foods. Second, a varied diet reduced in energy content remains highly palatable, thereby serving as a constant source of temptation to the dieter. Also, the calorie counting method tends to assume that obese persons exhibit an orderly pattern of eating and simply eat too much of certain meals. In point of fact, there is growing evidence that many obese individuals have poorly structured eating patterns, with some meals skipped, many snacks consumed, and occasional food binges.

As a result of increasing recognition of the ineffectiveness of this method of weight control, this method is now being rarely recommended.

VITAMIN B-6 (Pyridoxine)

Functions: Is essential in the metabolism of protein, all protein structures in the body from glands to blood vessels are dependent on B-6 sufficiency.

It is required for the production of anti-bodies for the immunological system. Requirement increased by protein intake.

A deficiency may result in irritability, convulsions and muscular twitching.

NATURAL SOURCES:

Meats, organ meats, whole grain cereals, soybeans, peanuts and wheat germ are rich sources. Milk and green vegetables supply smaller amounts.

VITAMIN B-12

FUNCTIONS: It is necessary for normal metabolism of nervous tissue and is involved in protein, fat and carbohydrate metabolism.

It is the only vitamin that contains essential mineral elements.

It aids in the absorption of iron.

It helps the placement of Vitamin A into body tissue.

A deficiency may result in pernicious anemia, neurologic disorders, and kidney stones.

NATURAL SOURCES:

Liver is the best source; kidney, muscle meats, fish and dairy products are other good sources. It is not present in plant foods in sufficient amounts to be considered a significant dietary source.

MULTI VITAMINS

Vitamins are a heterogeneous group of organic molecules required by the body for a variety of essential metabolic functions. Most of the water – soluble (B- complex) vitamins act as co-enzymes, or organic catalysts; the four fat soluble vitamins (A, D, E AND K) have more diverse functions. The intake of multi- vitamins is used as a prophylaxis against possible vitamin and mineral deficiency.

PLATEAUS:

Weight loss is not always linear, because the oxidation of body fat stores result in the production of equivalent amount of water. This water will accumulate in the body until released. If you comply with the program you have selected to do for your height, and body size then the plateau is your body adjusting to weight loss and you could be holding a little water.

Remember water weighs more than fat that was oxidized (approx. 14% more i.e. F.A. (fatty acids) weighs, 284 units and 1 H20 (water) weighs 324 units).

B-12 PRODUCT ADVANTAGES

Is an excellent product for vegetarians; who are usually deficient in B-12.

Many nutritionists believe B-12 is critical for the transport of oxygen.

Via hemoglobin-hence, helps increase energy levels.

Non-timed; release for rapid dissolution and assimilation.

Helps build red blood cells.

Contains; cobalt a necessary mineral.

Contains: no sugar, starch or preservatives.

And it is yeast free.

B-6 PRODUCT ADVANTAGES

It is water soluble.

It properly assimilates protein and fat.

It aides in the conversion of tryptophan, an essential amino acid to niacin.

It helps prevent various nervous and skin disorders.

It works as a natural diuretic.

It is necessary for converting amino acids into neuro-transmitters and important protein synthesis.

Vitamin B6 is important for women taking oral contraceptives.

It contains no sugar, starch or preservatives.

And it is yeast free.

Over the years working with women and weight loss thousands of us are deficient in the B vitamin. Through childbirth, stress, work, etc. my advice to all women over 40 is take a B- complex vitamin every day you can get them in B-50 or B-100s. Jameson's make a very good product start with the lower dose you should feel the effects in two weeks. Your body will let you know if you need more.

Just a little tip from me!

Women who are pregnant or breast feeding should not be dieting. You should be consuming well balanced diets.

If you have had a heart attack within the last six months you should not be dieting. If you are overweight wait until your doctor gives you the OK.

If you have had a stroke (cerebrovascular disease) or Transient Ischemic attack (TIA) within the last year, you should not be dieting. Diets may promote rapid fluid mobilization that could produce hypotension (low blood pressure) with subsequent hypo –perfusion of the brain. If you are overweight wait until your doctor gives you the OK.

Renal dysfunctions: if you have a history of renal failure, renal damage, single kidney, you should not be dieting.

Children under the age of 10 should not be dieting. If you have an overweight child follow the guidelines provided for you in this book.

Type 1 diabetes Mellitus should not be dieting. Follow the diabetic information provided in this book.

If you have or had an eating disorder (Bulimia/Anorexia) you should not be dieting. Follow the guideline that I have provided for you in this book.

MENOPAUSE

We all go through it; just like everything else here is a little over view for you. I hope it helps you out.

Premature menopause symptoms

In addition to dealing with hot flashes, mood swings, and other symptoms that accompany menopause, many women undergoing premature menopause have to cope with additional physical and emotional concerns.

Premature menopause is menopause that happens before the age of 40 whether it is natural or induced. Women who enter menopause early get symptoms similar to those of natural menopause, like hot flashes, emotional problems, vaginal dryness, and decreased sex drive.

Menopause is the end of a woman's menstrual cycle and fertility. It happens when the ovaries no longer make estrogen and progesterone, two hormones needed for a woman's fertility, and periods have stopped for 1 year.

The term menopause is commonly used to describe any of the changes a woman experiences either just before or after she stops menstruating, marking the end of reproductive period.

Menopause simply means the end of menstruating for one year. As a woman ages, there is a gradual decline in the function of her ovaries and the production of estrogen.

Some women experience induced menopause as a result of surgery or medical treatments, such as chemotherapy, and pelvic radiation therapy.

When menopause symptoms occur, they may include hot flashes, night sweats, pain during intercourse, increased anxiety or irritability and the need to urinate more often.

Millions of women with menopausal like symptoms, even those taking estrogen, may be suffering from undiagnosed thyroid disease. While symptoms such as fatigue, depression, mood swings, and sleep disturbances are frequently associated with menopause, they may also be signs of hypothyroidism.

Because hormone levels may fluctuate greatly in an individual woman, even from one day to the next, they are not a reliable indicator for diagnosing menopause.

The risk of breast cancer increases with age. That is why it is very important for all menopausal women to get regular mammograms.

Menopause is not linked to a higher risk of developing cancer. But the rates of many cancers, including ovarian cancer, do rise with age.

Having regular pelvic exams may help in early detection of certain cancers in both menopausal and postmenopausal women.

There is a direct relationship between the lack of estrogen after menopause and the contribution to osteoporosis. Because symptoms of osteoporosis may not develop until bone loss is extensive. It is important for woman at risk for osteoporosis to undergo regular bone testing.

Once a woman reaches the age of 50 about the age of natural menopause; her risk for heart disease increases dramatically. In young women who have undergone early or surgical menopause, who do not take estrogen, their risk for heart disease is also higher.

Fortunately, many of the signs and symptoms associated with

menopause are temporary. Here are some tips to help reduce or prevent their effects.

Dress in layers, have a cold glass of water or go somewhere cooler. Try to pinpoint what triggers your hot flashes. For many women, triggers may include hot beverages, caffeine, spicy foods, alcohol, stress, hot weather, and even a hot room.

Decrease vaginal discomfort use over the counter, water based vaginal lubricants (Astroglide, K-Y jelly etc.) or moisturizers choose products that do not contain glycerin, which can cause burning or irritation in women who are sensitive to that chemical. Staying sexually active also helps by increasing blood flow to the vagina. Get enough sleep, avoid caffeine, which can make it hard to get to sleep, and avoid drinking too much alcohol, which can interrupt sleep. Exercise during the day, not right before bedtime. If hot flashes disturb your sleep, you may have to find a way to manage them before you can get adequate rest. Techniques such as deep breathing, paced breathing, guided imagery, massage and progressive muscle relaxation can help relieve menopausal symptoms. Eat a balanced diet include a variety of fruits, vegetables, and whole grains, limit saturated fats, oils, and sugars.

Many women reject the risks associated with hormone replacement therapy to treat their menopause symptoms and instead seek relief from alternative sources; as menopausal women face fluctuating levels of estrogen and progesterone. Luckily, there's an array of natural remedies available to help you cope.

Do Mother Nature's Treatments Help Hot Flashes

Black Cohosh: (Actaea racemosa- Cimicifuga racemosa.) This herb has received quite a bit of scientific attention for its possible effects on hot flashes. Studies of its effectiveness in reducing hot flashes have produced mixed results. However, some women report that it has helped them. Recent research suggests that black cohosh does not act like estrogen, as once thought. This reduces concerns about its effect on hormone- sensitive tissue (e.g., uterus, breast) black cohosh has had a good safety record over a number of years. Although there have been reports linking black cohosh to liver problems, and this connection continues to be studied.

Red Clover: (Trifolium pratense): In five controlled studies, no consistent or conclusive evidence was found that red clover leaf extract reduces hot flashes. As with black cohosh, however, some women claim that red clover has helped them. Studies report few side effects and no serious health problems with use. But studies in animals have raised concerns that red clover might have harmful effects on hormone – sensitive tissue.

Dong Quai: (Angelica sinensis): has been used in traditional Chinese medicine to treat gynecologic conditions for more than 1,200 years. Yet only one randomized clinical study of dong quai has been conducted to determine its effects on hot flashes, and this botanical therapy was not found to be useful in reducing them. Some experts on Chinese medicine point out that the preparation studied was not the same as they use in practice. Dong Quai should never be used by women with fibroids or blood clotting problems such as hemophilia, or by women taking drugs that affect clotting such as warfarin (Coumadin) as bleeding complications can result.

Ginseng: (Panax ginseng or panax quinquefolius): Research has shown that ginseng may help with some menopausal symptoms, such as mood symptoms and sleep disturbances, and with one's overall sense of well-being. However, it has not been found to be helpful for hot flashes.

Kava: (Piper methysticum): may decrease anxiety, but there is no evidence that it decreases hot flashes. It is important to note that kava has been associated with liver disease. The FDA has issued a warning to patients and providers about kava because of its potential to damage the liver. Because of this concern, Health Canada does not allow it to be sold in Canada.

Evening primrose: (Oenothera biennis): This botanical is also promoted to relieve hot flashes. However, the only randomized, placebo- controlled study found no benefit over placebo (mock medication). Reported side effects include inflammation, problems with blood clotting and the immune system, nausea and diarrhea. It has been shown to induce seizures in patients diagnosed with schizophrenia who are taking antipsychotic medication. Evening primrose oil should not be use with anticoagulants or phenothiazine's (a type of psychotherapeutic agent).

Use with caution as with all therapies, there are some risks involved, the public usually takes herbal therapies in the form of supplement pills, not as a preparation made directly from the herb by a trained herbalist.

Keep in mind that herbal supplements are not as closely regulated as prescription drugs.

The amount of herbal product, quality, safety, and purity may vary between brands or even between batches of the same brand. Herbal therapies may also interact with prescription drugs, resulting in dramatic changes in the effect of the botanical, the drug, or both. To be safe talk to your doctor or health care provider about all botanical therapies you are considering and always stop all herbal treatments at least 2 weeks before any planned surgery.

The best way to look at menopause is that you are not alone millions of women are experiencing it right along with you.

When I was going through it I said to myself. This too will pass.

DIABETES

Glycemic index or (GI)

GI is a scale that ranks carbohydrate- rich foods by how much they raise blood glucose levels. GI helps with diabetes control. Foods with a low GI raise blood glucose levels more slowly than foods with a higher GI. Foods are compared against a standard food, white bread, or glucose, and ranked low, medium, or high GI. Foods with low GI include most vegetables and fruit, legumes, whole grain bread, pasta and milk. How food is prepared, what foods are eaten together, and the amount and type of carbohydrate eaten all affect blood glucose.

Many starch foods have a high GI. Choose low and medium foods more often.

Low GI less than (55) choose most often

Breads = 100% stoned ground whole wheat and pumpernickel

Cereal = ready to eat bran cereal, oatmeal, oat bran

Grains = parboiled or converted rice, barley and bulgur, pasta and noodles

Other =sweet potato/yam, legumes (lentils, chickpeas, kidney beans, split peas, soy beans, baked beans) 1% milk

Medium GI (56-70) choose more often

Breads = whole wheat, rye and pita

Cereals = partially cooked oats and cream of wheat

Grains = basmati rice, brown rice, and couscous

Other = new potato, sweet corn, popcorn, stoned wheat thins, crackers, black beans soup, green pea soup, and digestive biscuits

High GI (more than 70) choose less often

Breads = white bread, Kaiser Roll and bagels

Cereal = bran or cornflakes, crisp rice cereal and oat O cereal

Grains = short grain rice and brand rice

Other = baked potato, French fries, pretzels, rice cakes, and soda crackers

BLOOD SUGAR LEVELS= understanding and managing your highs and lows

Levels that are too high (hyperglycaemia) or too low (hypoglycaemia) can quickly turn into a diabetic emergency without quick and appropriate treatment. The best way to avoid dangerously high or low blood sugar levels is to self- test to stay in tune with your body and to stay attuned to the symptoms and risk factors for hypoglycaemia diabetic ketoacidosis and hyperosmolar (hyperglycaemia).

Low blood sugar emergencies (hypoglycaemia)

Hypoglycaemia is sometimes called “insulin reaction” because it is more frequent in people with diabetes who take insulin. However, it can occur in either type 1 or type 2 diabetes, and is also commonly caused by certain oral medications, missed meals, and exercise without proper precautions. The typical threshold for hypoglycaemia is 70 mg/dl. Although it may be higher or lower depending on a patients individual blood glucose target range. Symptoms include erratic heartbeat, sweating, dizziness, confusion, unexplained fatigue, shaking, hunger and potential loss of consciousness. Once a low is recognized it should be treated immediately with a fast acting carbohydrate such as glucose tablets or juice.

Hi blood sugar emergencies (DKA or HHNS)

Extremely high blood sugar levels can lead to one of two conditions – DKA (diabetic ketoacidosis) and hyperglycaemia nonketotic syndrome. (HHNS also called hyperglycaemia hyperosmolar nonketotic coma).

Although both syndromes can occur in either type 1 or type 2diabetes, DKA is more common in type 1 and HHNS is more common in type 2.

Type 1 diabetes also known as juvenile diabetes, insulin dependent diabetes (IDDM), childhood diabetes and ketosis prone diabetes type 1 diabetes accounts for between 5 and 10% of all diagnosed diabetes in the United States.

Although type 1 diabetes develops most often in children and young adults (one in every 400-600 children has type 1 diabetes) the disease can be diagnosed at any age throughout the lifespan, and is equally distributed among males and females. Type 2diabetes is more common in Caucasians than in those Latino, African American or other non-Caucasian backgrounds

Type 1 diabetes is an autoimmune disease that occurs when the insulin- producing beta cells within the pancreas are gradually destroyed and eventually fail to produce insulin. Insulin is a hormone that helps the body's cells use glucose for energy, blood glucose (or blood sugar) is manufactures from the food we eat (primarily carbohydrates) and by the liver. If glucose can't be absorbed by the cells, it builds up in the blood stream instead, and high blood sugar is the result. Over time the high blood glucose levels of uncontrolled diabetes can be toxic to virtually every system of the body.

Because type 1 diabetes is frequently diagnosed in childhood, effective management is important to prevent some of the more serious complications of diabetes, which include heart disease, blindness, stroke, nerve damage, and kidney failure. In addition to following a healthy eating plan and exercise, individuals with type 1 must receive insulin by injection or pump.

The causes of type 1 diabetes are complex and still not completely understood. People with type 1 are thought to have inherited or genetic predisposition to the disease. Researchers believe that this genetic predisposition may remain dormant until it is activated by an environmental trigger or triggers such as a virus or a chemical. This starts an attack of the immune system that results in the eventual destruction of the beta cells of the pancreas. There are several subtypes of type 1 diabetes the basic treatment is the same for all (insulin injections).

A so called diabetic diet is not a life sentence to a rigid and restrictive menu plan. There is not one ultimate diabetic diet that everyone should follow instead; nutritional management of diabetes is a lifestyle that balances moderation and healthy food choices.

When you have diabetes, you need to maintain fairly even blood sugar levels. This means that you need to eat three meals a day, and include some healthy snacks into your schedule. Try not to space your meals more than six hours apart.

Drink lots of water. If you reach for a can of pop or juice every time you get thirsty, you will raise your blood sugar level.

Try to avoid sugars and sweets such as soda, desserts, candy, jam and honey. These will raise your blood sugar levels.

Be smart when it comes to high fat foods, ask yourself if you really need the potato chips, pastries or fried food. High fat will cause you to gain weight, which will negatively impact your diabetes.

Maintaining a healthy weight helps your blood glucose levels, and it is good for your heart, whole grain foods are good for your heart, and they may help you feel fuller. This includes beans, whole grain breads and cereals and brown rice.

Fruits and vegetables are key to a healthy diet when you have diabetes because they provide not only whole grains but also important vitamins to keep your body running healthily. Fruits and vegetables are not only high in nutrients, but they are also low in calories.

Just like any diet, a diabetes diet is not complete unless you are also active; exercise is another key ingredient to helping you stay healthy.

When you plan your meal, mentally divide your plate into four sections. If you fill two of these sections with vegetables (try to have at least two kinds of vegetable at each meal), one with meat and one with a grain, you will be on the path to healthier eating immediately. If you drink a glass of milk with dinner, you will have covered all food groups. Eating a piece of fruit for dessert will nicely round out your meal.

It is important to eat a carbohydrate at each meal (the starch or grain part of dinner). These foods such as potatoes, rice, noodles or bread, are broken down into the energy that your body needs to function.

When you are choosing your protein, consider choosing a lean meat, fish or cottage cheese or vegetarian protein option to help keep your fat down.

One of the keys to diet is portion sizes, weigh and measure your food for a few weeks while you are getting used to monitoring your food intake. Remember a serving of meat is the size of the palm of your hand and the thickness of your baby finger. Whereas a serving of starch is the size of your fist; limit high fat intake and measure your vegetable servings by how much you can hold in both hands. If you drink alcohol, it will affect your blood sugar. Establish how much alcohol you can and should be drinking with your doctor

HEALTHY DIET PLAN FOR DIABETICS

Following a strict diet plan is very important for those who are diabetic. What many people don't know is that a diabetic diet plan is nearly the healthiest diet people can live by, whether they are suffering from diabetes or not.

The importance of having a diet plan

For diabetics, their diet plan is considered part of the treatment for their condition. Known as medical nutrition therapy (MNT), the diet helps keep the body from being overwhelmed by the things it can't handle efficiently, which are mainly sugar and carbohydrates that turn into sugar in the body. Diabetics also frequently have secondary health problems such as dyslipidemia and problems with the levels of cholesterol in the body. A healthy diet plan is essential for managing blood sugar and maintaining a healthy weight, which is often a problem for diabetics.

When a diabetic eats excess amounts of fat, carbohydrates and calories, the body responds with a dangerous rise in blood sugar. Over time this can lead to chronic health concerns such as nerve, kidney and heart damage. In fact diabetes and its complications play a role in more than 231,000 deaths each year, so maintaining a healthy diet is essential.

Those with type 2 diabetes; often find that the diet required to keep their diabetes stable is also a healthy way to keep their weight under control, since type 2 is often the result of obesity. There are some foods that are great for the body and they should definitely be included in a diabetic diet plan. When it comes to a MNT diet plan the quality of what is eaten is just as important as the quality.

FIBER- works like a broom in the cardiovascular system to help rid the body of excess cholesterol, as well as absorbing water in the digestive tract to ensure that it is functioning properly. Fiber also doesn't cause the wild blood sugar spikes that other forms of carbohydrates do.

The advantage of the following fibers is that they are known to reduce the risk of obesity, cut down on blood-sugar swings, and reduce heart disease, bowel disorders and cancer. There are six forms of fiber each with a function of its own. You should start with small amounts of fiber and gradually increase your intake until the stools are the proper consistency.

Pectin – is good for diabetics because it slows down food absorption after meals, removes unwanted metals and toxins, pectin is valuable during treatment with radiation therapy or x rays, and it helps lower cholesterol, lessens the risk of heart disease and gallstones. Pectin is found in apples, carrots, beets, bananas, the cabbage family, the citrus family, in dried peas and okra.

Cellulose – good for hemorrhoids, varicose veins, colitis and diverticulitis; it is excellent for removal of cancer-causing substances from the colon wall, constipation and a boost for weight loss. Cellulose is found in apples, pears, the cabbage family, carrots, broccoli, lima beans, peas, whole grains, Brazil nuts, green beans and beets.

Hemicellulose – good for weight loss, constipation and colon cancer, it fights carcinogens in the intestinal tract. Hemicellulose is found in apples, beets, whole grain cereals, cabbage, Brussel sprouts, bananas, green beans, corn, peppers, broccoli, mustard greens and pears.

Lignin – good for lowering cholesterol levels, protecting against colon cancer and preventing gall stone formation. It binds with bile acids to remove them. It's recommended for diabetics. Lignin is found in the cabbage family (cauliflower, etc.) carrots, green beans, peas, whole grains, Brazil nuts, peaches, tomatoes, strawberries and potatoes.

Gums & mucilage – they regulate blood glucose levels, aid in lowering cholesterol levels and help in the removal of toxins. These are found in oatmeal, oat bran, sesame seeds and dried beans. Fiber helps to remove fat from the colon wall and unwanted metals and toxins from our bodies. In today's polluted environment our bodies need help in excreting this overload. Increase your intake of raw foods and supplement your diet with extra fiber.

Healthy carbs- not all carbs are created equal. The sugars that a person eats are called simple carbs. The starches that a person eats are called complex carbs. Both types of carbs break down in the body into blood glucose, but the more processed the carbs are (such as white flour or white sugar) the faster they will break down, which means the body will experience a spike in blood glucose, he healthiest carbs are those that are the least processed and contain fiber such as fruits, vegetables, whole grains, legumes and dairy. These also provide the majority of the nutrients that the body needs to be healthy.

Heart healthy protein- the best forms of protein are chicken and fish. Both are lower in saturated fat and cholesterol, where fish, in particular, is rich in omega- 3 fatty acids that aid in heart health by lowering triglycerides. This is important because triglyceride levels tend to be quite high in diabetics. Chicken should be served without skin and baked, broiled, or grilled to avoid consuming excess fat. Most types of fish are considered healthy, but the best are salmon, mackerel and herring because they are highest in omega-3 fatty acids. People should be careful though because there can be concerns about high levels of mercury in some fish.

Good fat- is those that help lower cholesterol such as monounsaturated fats and polyunsaturated fats. These include foods like avocado, nuts, olives and certain oils. Diabetics still need to be careful when using the, however, because all fats contain a large amount of calories.

Because diabetes increases the risk for cardiovascular disease, there are some things that diabetics need to avoid- cholesterol such as that from full fat dairy, animal based protein, organ meat, eggs and shellfish should be consumed sparingly. Saturated fats such as that found in full fat dairy products, beef, deli meats and pork products should also be consumed sparingly. Tran's fat such as those found in processed foods, shortening and stick margarine should be completely avoided. Sodium is important to several functions of the body, but too much can cause problems such as high blood pressure, congestive heart failure, liver and kidney problems, heart attack and stroke. A healthy diet plan isn't just good for diabetics, it's good for everyone. The improved health that follows will surely be worth the effort.

Diabetes how to control blood sugar levels:

If you're living with diabetes, you don't have to deprive yourself of certain types of food. In fact, all foods can fit into your diabetes meal plan;

as long as you find the right balance between how often you eat them and the proper portion size.

Furthermore, diabetes meal plans can work for the entire family. So if you're caring for someone who has the disease you don't have to make separate meals.

Get to know your carbohydrates, proteins and fats; what you may not realize is that all foods- from baked apples to baked ziti – break down into a combination of carbohydrates, proteins and fats. All carbohydrates are not created equal, so the glycemic index (GI) rating – like whole grain breads, yams, and legumes. For people living with diabetes, it's especially important to consume low (GI) foods that won't send blood sugar levels soaring. When setting meal plans and grocery shopping, try to select foods that are close to their natural state- like raw fruits and vegetables, converted and parboiled rice and whole grain breads and cereals.

Proteins – your body needs proteins to build and maintain tissue. The good news is that meat, fish, poultry. Shell fish and other proteins don't have a significant impact on blood sugar levels. But they do contain calories. Studies have shown a link between obesity and type 2 diabetes. According to the Canadian diabetes association, even moderate weight loss can be beneficial to your health.

Fat- like proteins, fats will not significantly impact blood sugar levels, and they are necessary for the healthy functioning of your vital organs. But all types of fat contain a great number of calories. Not surprisingly, fat contains more calorie than proteins and carbohydrates. It's important to limit your consumption of fats. You should also pay close attention to the types of fat you eat.

Look for products low in saturated and Tran's fats- like low fat dairy products and lean cuts of meat.

Go easy on the butter, margarine and salad dressing. Use low fat cooking methods like steaming, grilling and roasting. Stay away from anything labelled "hydrogenated".

Controlling the types and amount of fat you eat can help control your weight and make it easier to manage your diabetes.

Spread meals and snacks throughout the day; perhaps three meals a day suits you just fine.

Or maybe your preference is for three meals plus snacks; whether you snack or not, if you have diabetes it's important to spread your meals throughout the day, as this will help regulate your blood sugar levels and prevent peaks and valleys.

It's also important to remember that snacking can easily add extra carbohydrates and calories, which can negatively impact your blood sugar levels and weight.

When you snack, you need to reduce the size of your regular meals, so you don't overeat

Type 2 diabetes is a complex disease: many variables can make type2 diabetes difficult to control. Healthy food choices are only one part of a good diabetes management strategy.

Healthy living can prevent or delay the onset of type 2 diabetes since genetic risk factors are associated with type 2 diabetes, it's important to instil the principles of healthy living in your children or grandchildren. By teaching them early on to make proper food choices and to exercise regularly, you can help reduce their risk of developing type2 diabetes later in life. Remember healthy eating doesn't have to be boring. Choose healthier fats, and use less of them.

Reduce your consumption of sugar. Select low GI foods (e.g., sweet potatoes) over their high GI counterparts (e.g. white potatoes)

The good news is that diabetes doesn't mean giving up all your favourite foods or avoiding sugar entirely. The nutrition basics for people with diabetes apply to everyone, so practicing the tips below can benefit you and your family too.

Go for fibre: select nutrient rich carbohydrates like whole grains, fruit, vegetables, beans and other legumes. These foods have fibre, which is useful in helping to keep blood sugar in control.

The facts about fat: eating less fat overall is important for maintaining a healthy weight and in reducing your risk of heart disease. Most importantly, choose foods that are low in saturated fat and are Trans- fat free; it is easier than ever to cut back on fat with the growing variety of great tasting food choices in grocery stores by making lower fat food choices you not only limit total fat intake but also saturated and Trans-fat, cholesterol and often calories. Read nutrition facts panels and watch out for low-fat foods that replace fat with sugar. Foods with no added sugar can help; even though foods with sugar can fit into a well- balanced diet, foods and beverages with no add sugar are great choices for managing diabetes. They generally have fewer carbohydrates per serving and some are also lower in calories. It is important to note that products with no added sugar may contain naturally occurring sugars that will still affect your blood sugar. For example "100% fruit juice with no sugar added" will still contain sugar from the fruit that it's made with. Having diabetes does not mean having to avoid any particular food – especially desert! To have good blood sugar control, you may need to limit the amount of total carbohydrates you eat, but the good news is that you can still eat sweet food in moderation. This is because it is the amount of carbohydrate that has more of an impact on blood glucose rather than the type of carbohydrate (sugar vs. starches).

GESTATIONAL DIABETES AND PREGNANCY

Protein equivalents
Food
1 cup milk=8 grams protein
1 cup plain yogurt = 8 grams protein
1oz American processed cheese = 7 grams protein
1oz cheese = 7 grams protein
1 tbsp. peanut butter = 7 grams protein
¼ cup cottage cheese = 7 grams protein
½ cup cooked dried beans = 7 grams protein
1 slice whole wheat bread = 3 grams protein
½ cup flaked cereal bran or corn = 3 grams protein

The daily need for calories increases by 300 calories during the second and third trimesters of pregnancy. If non pregnant calorie intake was 1800 calories per day and weight was maintained, a calorie intake of 2100 calories per day from 14 weeks until delivery. This is the equivalent of an additional 8 ounce glass of 2% milk and one half of a sandwich 1 slice of bread, approximately 1oz meat, and a teaspoon of butter etc. per day.

The need for protein also increases during pregnancy. Make sure your diet includes foods high in protein, but not in fat. Most vitamins and minerals are also needed in larger amounts during pregnancy. This can be attained by increasing dairy products; especially those low in fat, and make sure you include whole grain cereals and breads as well as fruits and vegetables in your diet each day.

To make sure you get enough folate (a B vitamin critical during pregnancy) and iron, your obstetrician will probably recommend a prenatal vitamin. Prenatal vitamins do not replace a good diet; they merely help you to get the nutrients you need. To absorb the most iron from your prenatal vitamin, take it at night before going to bed, or in the morning on an empty stomach.

The daily food guide serves as a guideline for food sources that provide important vitamins and minerals, as well as carbohydrates, protein, and fibre during pregnancy.

The recommended mineral servings per day appear in parenthesis after each food group listed. This guide emphasizes foods that are low in fat and sugar.

Daily food guide for gestational diabetes and pregnancy

Each item equals one serving.

Milk and milk products = 4 servings daily. 1 cup milk or 1 ½oz cheese (high protein, calcium and vitamin D)

Meat and poultry substitutes = 5-6 servings daily. 1oz cooked poultry, fish or lean meat (beef, lamb, pork) 1 tbsp. peanut butter, 1 egg, ¼ cup cottage cheese, ½ cup cooked dried beans or lentils. (High protein B vitamin and iron)

Starches = 5-6 servings daily. 1slice whole grain bread, 5 crackers, 1 muffin, biscuit, pancake, or waffle, ¾ cup dried cereal unsweetened.

High complex carbohydrates = ½ cup pasta, (macaroni, spaghetti), rice, mashed potatoes, or cooked cereal. 1/3 cup sweet potato or yams, ½ cup cooked dried beans or lentils, ½ bagel, ½ muffin or flour tortillas. 1 small baked potato, 2taco shells= (a good source of protein, B-vitamins, fibre and minerals)

Fresh fruit or frozen = 2 servings daily: ½ banana or 1 medium sized fruit (apple, orange, ½ cup orange, grapefruit, or fresh mixed fruit fortified with vitamin C.

1 cup strawberries, ½ cup fresh apricots, nectarines, purple plums, cantaloupe or 4 halves dried apricots=(vitamin A source) fresh fruit provides fibre; (include one Vitamin C source daily).

Vegetables = 2 servings daily: ½ cup cooked or 1 cup raw broccoli, spinach, carrots, (vitamin A source) 1/3 cup mixed vegetables (include good vitamin A sources at least every other day).

Fats = 2 servings daily 1 tsp butter or margarine, 1 tsp oil or mayonnaise, 1 tbsp. regular salad dressing or ¼ cup nuts or seeds.

1oz cheese can be used as 1 serving from the meat, poultry, fish and meat substitutes group if sufficient calcium is already being provided from 4 meat servings. This refers to plain yogurt; commercially fruited yogurt contains a lot of added sugar. Starchy vegetables such as corn, peas, and potatoes are included in breads, cereals, and other starches.

The food guide is divided into six groups: milk and milk products, meats, poultry, fish and meat substitutes, breads, cereal and other starches, fruits, vegetables, and fats. Each group provides its own combination of vitamins minerals and other nutrients which play an important part in nutrition during pregnancy.

Omitting the foods from one group will leave your diet inadequate in other nutrients. Plan your meals using a variety of foods within each food group, in the amounts recommended and you'll be more likely to get all the vitamins and minerals and other nutrients the fetus needs for growth and development.

The following outlines food patterns which help to keep blood sugar levels within acceptable range.

Avoid foods high in sugar. Most women with gestational diabetes just like those without have a desire for something sweet in their diet.

In pregnant women sugar is rapidly absorbed into the blood and requires a larger release of insulin to maintain normal blood sugar levels.

Without the larger release of insulin, blood sugar levels will increase excessively when you eat sugar containing foods.

There are many forms of sugar such as table sugar, honey, brown sugar, corn syrup and molasses generally food that ends in "ose" is a sugar(e.g. sucrose, dextrose and glucose).

Foods that usually contain high amounts of sugar include pies, cakes, cookies, ice cream, candy, soft drinks, fruit drinks, fruit packed in syrup, commercially fruited yogurt, jams, jelly, doughnuts and sweet rolls. Many of these are high in fat as well.

Fruit juices should only be taken with a meal and limited to 6 ounces. Tomato juice is a good choice as it is lower in sugar; six ounces of most other juice (apple, grapefruit, and orange) with no sugar added still contain approximately 4 to 5 teaspoons of sugar. However, these do not contain much of the fibre of a piece of fruit which normally would act to slow the absorption of sugar into the blood. If you drink juice frequently to quench your thirst during the day, a high blood sugar may result. Use only whole fruit for snacks. Drink water.

Sample menu – 2000 calories
Breakfast
½ grapefruit
¾ cup oatmeal, cooked
1 tsp raisins
1 whole wheat English muffin
1 tsp butter or margarine

Lunch
Salad with
1 cup romaine lettuce
½ cup kidney beans, cooked
½ fresh tomato
1oz mozzarella cheese
2 tbsp. Italian dressing
½ cup cantaloupe chunks

Afternoon snack
2 rice cakes
6oz plain yogurt
½ cup blueberries

Dinner
1tsp butter or margarine
¾ cup vegetable soup with
¼ cup cooked barley
3oz chicken breast, skin removed
1 baked potato
½ cup cooked broccoli

1 slice whole wheat bread

Bedtime snack
1 apple
2 cups popcorn plain 1 tsp butter or margarine
¼ cup peanuts

VEGETARIANISM: is the practice of abstaining from the consumption of meat (red meat, poultry, seafood and the flesh of any other animal), and may include abstention from by-products of animal slaughter.

Vegetarianism can be adopted for different reasons. Many object to eating meat out of respect for sentient life. Such ethical motivations have been codified under various religious beliefs, along with animal rights. Other motivations for vegetarianism are health- related, political, environmental, cultural, aesthetic, economic, or personal preference. There are varieties of the diet as well: ovo-vegetarian diet includes eggs but not dairy products, a lacto- vegetarian diet includes dairy products but not eggs, and an ovo- lacto vegetarian diet includes both eggs and dairy products. A vegan diet excludes all animal products, including eggs, dairy, and honey. Some vegans also avoid other animal products such as beeswax, leather or silk clothing, and goose – fat shoe polish.

Various packaged or processed foods, including cake, cookies, candies, chocolate, yogurt and marshmallows, often contain unfamiliar ingredients, and may be a special concern for vegetarians due to the likelihood of such additions.

Often, products are reviewed by vegetarians for animal- derived ingredients prior to purchase or consumption. Vegetarians vary in their feelings regarding these ingredients, however. For example, while some vegetarians may be unaware of animal-derived rennet's role in the usual production of cheese and may therefore unknowingly consume the product; other vegetarians may not take issue with its consumption.

Semi vegetarian diets consist largely of vegetarian foods, but may include fish or poultry, or sometimes other meats, on and infrequent basis. Those with diets containing fish or poultry may define meat only as mammalian flesh and may identify with vegetarianism. A pescetarian diet has been described as "fish but no other meat". The common use association between such diets and vegetarianism has led vegetarian groups such as the vegetarian society to state that diets containing these ingredients are not vegetarian, because fish and birds are also animals.

There are a number of vegetarian diets, which exclude or include various foods.

Buddhist vegetarianism: Different Buddhist traditions have differing teachings on diet, which may also vary for ordained monks and nuns compared to others. Many interpret the precept "not to kill" to require abstinence from meat, but not all.

In Taiwan, su vegetarianism excludes not only all animal products nut also vegetables in the allium family (which have the characteristic aroma of onion and garlic): onion, garlic, scallions, leeks, chives, or shallots.

Fruitarians' permits only fruit, nuts, seeds, and other plant matter that can be gathered without harming the plant.

Jain vegetarianism includes dairy but excludes eggs and honey, as well as root vegetables.

Macrobiotic diets consist mostly of whole grains and beans.

Lacto vegetarianism includes dairy products but not eggs.

Ovo vegetarianism includes eggs but not dairy products.

Ovo – lacto vegetarianism (or lacto-ovo vegetarianism) includes animal/dairy products such as eggs, milk, and honey.

Sattvic diets (also known as yogic diet), a plant based diet which may also include dairy (not eggs) and honey, but excludes anything from the onion or leek family, red lentils, durian fruit, mushrooms, blue cheese, fermented foods or sauces, alcoholic drinks and often also excludes coffee, black or green tea, chocolate, nutmeg or any other type of stimulant such as excess sharp spices.

Veganism excludes all animal flesh and by-products, such as milk, honey, and eggs, as well as items refined or manufactured through any such product, such as bone – char refined white sugar or animal- tested baking soda.

Raw veganism includes only fresh and uncooked fruit, nuts, seeds, and vegetables. Vegetables can only be cooked up to a certain temperature, for instance using a dehydrator.

Some vegetarians also avoid products that may use animal ingredients not included on their labels oh which use animal products in their manufacturing; for example, sugars that are whitened with bone char, cheeses that use animal rennet (enzymes from animal stomach lining), gelatin (derived from the collagen inside animals' skin, bones and connective tissue), some cane sugar (but not beet sugar) and apple juice/ alcohol clarified with gelatin or crushed shellfish and sturgeon, while other vegetarians are unaware of or do not mind such ingredients.

Individuals sometimes label themselves "vegetarian" while practicing a semi-vegetarian diet; some dictionary definitions describe vegetarianism as sometimes including the consumption of fish, or only include mammalian flesh as part of their definition of meat, while other definitions exclude fish and all animal flesh.

In other cases, individuals may describe themselves as "flexitarian". These diets may be followed by those who reduce animal flesh consumed as a way of transitioning to a complete vegetarian diet or for health, ethical, environmental, or other reasons.

Semi – vegetarian diets include:

Macrobiotic diet: consisting mostly of whole grains and beans but can sometimes include fish.

Pescetarianism: which includes; fish and other forms of seafood.

"Pollo-pescetarian": This includes poultry and fish, or "white meat" only.

Pollotarianism: This includes chicken and possibly other poultry.

Semi- vegetarianism is contested by vegetarian groups, which states that vegetarianism excludes all animal flesh.

Health effects: compared to omnivores, vegetarian populations have a lower overall mortality rate and in particular benefit from a reduced incidence of many non- communicable diseases including heart disease, type 2diabetes and cerebrovascular disease. A vegetarian diet reduces cancer risk, except for breast cancer.

A vegetarian diet which is poorly planned can lead to hyperhomocysteinemia and platelet disorders; this risk may be offset by ensuring sufficient consumption of vitamin B-12 and polyunsaturated fatty acids.

Vegetarian diet offer lower levels of saturated fat, cholesterol and animal protein, and higher levels of carbohydrates, fibre, magnesium, potassium, folate, and antioxidants such as vitamins G and E and phytochemicals.

Vegetarian diets can meet guidelines for the treatment of diabetes and some research suggests that diets that are more plant- based reduce risk of type-2diabetes. Among possible explanations for a protective effect of vegetarian diets are the lower BMI of vegetarians and higher fiber intake of which improve insulin sensitivity.

Nutrition: vegetarian diets are typically high in carotenoids, but relatively low in omega-3 fatty acids and vitamin B-12. Vegans can have particularly low intake of vitamin B and calcium if they do not eat enough items such as collard greens, leafy greens, tempeh and tofu (soy). High levels of dietary fiber, folic acid, vitamins C and E, and magnesium, and low consumption of saturated fat are all considered to be beneficial aspects of a vegetarian diet. A well planned vegetarian diet will provide all nutrients in a meat – eater's diet to the same level for all stages of life.

Protein: intake in vegetarian diets is lower than in meat diets but can meet the daily requirements for most people. Studies in various countries confirmed that a vegetarian diet provides sufficient protein intake as long as a variety of plant sources are available and consumed. Pumpkin seeds, peanut butter, hemp seed, almonds, pistachio nuts, flaxseed, tofu, oats, soybeans, walnuts, are great sources of protein for vegetarians. Proteins are composed of amino acids, and a common concern with protein acquired from vegetable sources is an adequate intake of the essential amino acids, which cannot be synthesised by the human body. While dairy and egg products provide complete sources for ovo-lacto vegetarian, several vegetable sources have significant amounts of all eight types of essential amino acids, including lupin beans, soy, hempseed, chia seed, amaranth, buckwheat, pumpkin seeds, spirulina, pistachios, and quinoa.

However, the essential amino acids can also be obtained by eating a variety of complementary plant sources that, in combination, provide all eight essential amino acids(brown rice and beans, hummus and whole wheat pita, though protein combining in the same meal is not necessary).

Iron: vegetarian diets typically contain similar levels of iron to non-vegetarian diets, but this has low bioavailability than iron from meat sources, and its absorption can sometimes be inhibited by other dietary constituents. Consuming food that contains vitamin C, such as citrus fruit or juices, tomatoes or broccoli, is a good way to increase the amount of iron absorbed at a meal. Vegetarian foods rich in iron include black beans, cashews, hempseed, kidney beans, broccoli, lentils, oatmeal, raisins, spinach, cabbage, lettuce, black eyed peas, soybeans, many breakfast cereals, sunflower seeds, chickpeas, tomato juice, tempeh, molasses, thyme and whole wheat bread. The related vegan diets can often be higher in iron than vegetarian diets, because dairy products are low in iron. Iron stores often tend to be lower in vegetarians than non- vegetarians; and a few studies report very high rates of iron deficiency (up to 40% and 58% of the respective vegetarian or vegan groups). However iron deficiency is no-more common in vegetarians than non-vegetarians (adult males are rarely iron deficient); iron deficiency anaemia is rare no matter the diet.

Vitamin B -12 is not generally present in plants and is naturally found in foods of animal origin. Lacto – ovo vegetarians can obtain B-12 from dairy products and eggs, and vegans can obtain it from fortified foods (including some soy products and some breakfast cereals) and dietary supplements. Vitamin B -12 can also be obtained from fortified yeast extract products.

The recommended dietary allowance of B-12 per day 0.4 mcg (0-6 months), rising to 1.8 mcg (9-13 years), 2.4 mcg (14 + years), and 2.8 mcg (lactating female). While the body's daily requirement for vitamin B-12 is very small, deficiency of the vitamin is very serious leading to anemia and irreversible nerve damage.

Fatty acids: plant based or vegetarian sources of Omega 3 fatty acids include soy, walnuts, pumpkin seeds, canola oil, kiwifruit, hempseed, algae, chia seed, flaxseed, echium seed and leafy vegetables such as lettuce, spinach, cabbage, and purslane. Purslane contains more Omega 3 than any other known leafy green. Olives and olive oil are another important plant source of unsaturated fatty acids. Plant foods can provide alpha- linoleic acid which the human body uses to synthesize the long-chain n-3 fatty acids EPA. and DHA. can be obtained directly; in high amounts from oily fish or fish oils. Vegetarians, and particularly vegans, have lower levels of EPA. and DHA. Than those who eat meat.

Calcium intake in vegetarians and vegans can be similar to non-vegetarians, as long as the diet is properly planned. Lacto-ovo vegetarians that include dairy products can still obtain calcium from dairy sources, like milk, yogurt and cheese. Non- dairy milks that are fortified with calcium, such as soymilk, and almond milk can also contribute a significant amount of calcium in the diet.

The calcium found in broccoli, bok Choy and kale have also been found to have calcium that is well absorbed in the body. Though the calcium content per serving is lower in these vegetables than a glass of milk, the absorption of the calcium into the body is higher. Other foods that contain calcium include: calcium-set tofu, blackstrap molasses, turnip greens, mustard greens, soybeans, tempeh, almonds, okra, dried figs, and tahini. Although calcium can be found in spinach, Swiss chard, beans and beet greens, they are not considered to be a good source since the calcium binds to oxalic acid and is poorly absorbed into the body. Phytic acid found in nuts, seeds, and beans may also impact calcium absorption rates.

Vitamin D needs can be met via the human body's own generation upon sufficient and sensible exposure to the sun. Products including milk, soy milk, and cereal grains may be fortified to provide a source of Vitamin D. for those who do not get adequate sun exposure or food sources, Vitamin D supplementation may be necessary.

The key to a healthy vegetarian diet like any diet is to include a variety of foods. No single food can provide all the nutrients your body needs.

Healthy vegetarian eating pattern

Recommended servings for 2,000 calorie/day diet

Food groups = vegetables = 2 ½ cups daily, dark green 1 ½ cups per week,

Red and orange = 5 ½ cups per week,

Legumes (beans and peas) = 3 cups per week, or starchy = 5 cups per week,

Fruits = 2 cups per day,

Whole grains = 3 ½ ounces per day, Refined grains = 3 ounces per day,

Dairy = 3 cups per day

Protein foods = 3 ½ ounces per day

Meat, poultry, fish and eggs = 3 ounces per week

Nuts, seeds, soy products = 14 ounces per week

Added sugars, solid fats, added refined starches = no more than 290 calories a day (15% of total calories).

Keep in mind that the more restrictive your diet is, the more challenging it can be to get all the nutrients you need. A vegan diet, for example, eliminates natural food sources of vitamin B12, as well as milk products, which are good sources of calcium.

To be sure that your diet includes everything your body needs, pay special attention to the following nutrients:

Calcium and vitamin D – calcium helps build and maintain strong teeth and bones. Milk and dairy foods are highest in calcium. However, dark green vegetables, such as turnip and collard greens, kale and broccoli, are good plant sources when eaten in sufficient quantities. Calcium enriched and fortified products, including juices, cereals, soy milk, soy yogurt and tofu are other options.

Vitamin D also plays an important role in bone health. Vitamin D is added to cow's milk, some brands of soy and rice milk, and some cereals and margarines, be sure to check food labels. If you don't eat enough fortified foods and have limited sun exposure, you may need vitamin D supplement (one derived from plants)

Vitamin B-12 is necessary to produce red blood cells and prevent anemia. This vitamin is found almost exclusively in animal products, so it can be difficult to get enough B-12 on a vegan diet. Vitamin B-12 deficiency may go undetected in people who eat a vegan diet. This is because the vegan diet is rich in a vitamin called folate, which may mask deficiency in vitamin B-12 until severe problems occur. For this reason, it is important for vegans to consider vitamin supplements, vitamin – enriched cereals and fortified soy products.

Protein helps maintain healthy skin, bones, muscles and organs. Eggs and dairy products are good sources, and you don't need to eat large amounts to meet your protein needs. You can also get sufficient protein from plant-based foods if you eat a variety of them throughout the day. Plant sources include soy products and meat substitutes, legumes, lentils, nuts, seeds, and whole grains.

Omega-3 fatty acids are important for heart health. Diets that do not include fish and eggs are generally low in active forms of omega-3 fatty acids. Canola oil, soy oil, walnuts, ground flaxseed and soybeans are good sources of essential fatty acids. However, because conversion of plant-based omega – 3 to the types used by humans is inefficient, you may want to consider fortified products or supplements or both.

Iron and Zinc: Iron is a crucial component of red blood cells. Dried beans and peas, lentils, enriched cereals, whole-grain products, dark leafy green vegetables and dried fruits are good sources of iron. Because iron isn't as easily absorbed from plant sources, the recommended intake of iron for vegetarians is almost double that recommended for non-vegetarians. To help your body absorb iron, eat foods rich in vitamin C, such as strawberries, citrus fruits, tomatoes, cabbage and broccoli, at the same time as you're eating iron-containing foods.

Like iron, zinc is not as easily absorbed from plant sources as it is from animal products. Plant sources of zinc include whole grains, soy products, legumes, nuts and wheat germ. Zinc is an essential component of many enzymes and plays a role in cell division and in formation of proteins.

Iodine is a component in thyroid hormones, which help regulate metabolism, growth, and function of key organs. Vegans may not get enough iodine and may be at risk of deficiency and possibly even goiter. In addition, foods such as soybeans, cruciferous vegetables and sweet potato may promote a goiter. However, just ¼ teaspoon of iodized salt a day provides a significant amount of iodine.

One way to transition to a vegetarian diet is to gradually reduce the meat in your diet while increasing fruits and vegetables.

Ramp up: each week increase the number of meatless meals you already enjoy, such as spaghetti with tomato sauce or vegetable stir fry. Find ways to include greens, such as spinach, kale, chard and collards, in your daily meals.

Substitute: take favorite recipes and try them without meat. For example, make vegetarian chili by leaving out the ground beef and adding black beans. Or make fajitas using extra-firm tofu rather than chicken. You may be surprised to find that many dishes require only simple substitutions.

Branch out: buy or borrow vegetarian cookbooks, check out ethnic restaurants to sample vegetarian cuisines. To me variety is the spice of life, and the more you mix it up, the more likely you will be able to meet all your nutritional needs.

Healthy eating for vegans:

A vegan diet includes grains, vegetables, fruit, legumes (dried beans, peas and lentils), seeds and nuts. It excludes meat, fish, poultry, dairy and eggs and products containing these foods.

A healthy vegan diet has many health benefits including lower rates of obesity, heart disease, high blood pressure, high blood cholesterol, type 2 diabetes and certain types of cancer.

It may take planning to get enough protein, iron zinc, calcium, vitamin D, B 12, and omega- 3 fats from foods or supplements. A healthy vegan diet can meet all your nutrient needs at any stage of life including when you are pregnant, breast feeding, or for older adults.

Protein: is important for building and keeping muscles and red blood cells healthy. It supports growth all through the life cycle.

Sources of protein: soy and soy products like tofu, tempeh and fortified soy beverages, meat alternatives like textured vegetable protein and veggie burgers, dried beans (kidney, black and white beans), peas (chickpeas and black-eyed peas) and lentils (red, brown and green lentils) grains (quinoa, brown rice, bulgur and oatmeal), nuts, nut butters (hazelnuts and almond butter), and seeds (sesame and sunflower), peanuts and peanut butter.

Iron: helps carry oxygen to different parts of the body. Vegans need about twice as much dietary iron as non – vegetarians because the iron from plant foods (non – heme iron) is not as well absorbed as the iron from animal foods (heme iron). To meet these needs, vegans should choose iron-rich foods daily. Good sources of non-heme iron include: soy and soy products like firm tofu, tempeh, and fortified soy beverages. Meat alternatives like textured vegetable protein and veggie burgers, dried beans, peas and lentils like kidney, pinto and adzuki beans, chickpeas, and black-eyed peas, and red, brown and green lentils, fortified grain products (breads, cereals, and pasta), some nuts and seeds like cashews, almonds, pumpkin and sesame seeds, prune juice and dried apricots, vegetables like cooked spinach, kale and potatoes with their skins, and black strap molasses. Iron from vegetarian sources is better absorbed when eaten with vitamin – C rich foods.

Examples of vitamin C – rich foods include oranges and grapefruit and their juices, lemons, limes, kiwis, mangos, cantaloupe, potatoes, sweet peppers, broccoli, snow peas, and some green leafy vegetables.

Vitamin B-12: is important for making red blood cells and helping the body use fats. Good sources of vitamin B-12 include: red star nutritional yeast, fortified soy beverages and other fortified non-dairy beverages like rice and almond beverage, fortified meat alternatives like textured vegetable protein (TVP), veggie burgers and meatless chicken, fish and meatballs.

The number of servings needed daily of each group depends on your age, body size, activity level, whether you are male or female and if you are pregnant or breastfeeding.

Teens ages 13 to 18 years - grains = 6. Proteins = 6. Vegetables = 4. Fruit = 2.

Fats = 2. Calcium rich foods = 10.

Adults 19 years and older - grains =6. Proteins = 5. Vegetables = 4. Fruit = 2.

Fats = 2. Calcium rich foods = 8.

Pregnancy - grains = 6. Proteins = 7. Vegetables = 4. Fruit = 2. Fats = 2. Calcium rich foods = 8.

Breastfeeding - grains = 6. Proteins = 8. Vegetables = 4. Fruit = 2. Fats = 2.

Calcium rich foods = 8.

An example to serving size = 1 cup calcium fortified orange juice counts as 2 servings of fruit.

1 cup of fortified soymilk counts as 2 serving's legumes, nuts, and other protein-rich foods and 2 servings' calcium-rich foods.

2 slices of whole wheat toast counts as 2 servings of grain

2 tablespoons peanut butter counts as 1 serving legumes, nuts and other

Protein – rich foods.

FOOD GUIDE FOR VEGETARIANS

Calcium –rich foods = 8 to 10 servings daily

Grains Serving size

Whole wheat bread 1 slice

Cooked grain or cereal ½ cup (125ml)

Ready to eat cereal 1oz

Calcium fortified breakfast cereal 1oz

Legumes, Nuts and other protein –rich foods = 5 to 8 servings daily

Serving size

Cooked beans, peas or lentils ½ cup (125 ml)

Tofu or tempeh ½ cup (125 ml)

Nuts or seed butter 2 tbsp. (30 ml)
Nuts ¼ cup (60 ml)
Meat analog 1oz (28 g)
Egg 1
Cow's milk or yogurt or fortified soymilk ½ cup (125 ml)
Cheese ¾oz (21g)
Tempeh or calcium set tofu ½ cup (125 ml)
Almonds ¼ cup (60ml)
Almond butter or sesame tahini 2 tbsp. (30 ml)
Cooked soybeans ½ cup (125 ml)
Soy-nuts ¼ cup (60ml)

Vegetables = 4 servings daily
Cooked vegetables ½ cup (125ml)
Raw vegetables 1 cup (250 ml)
Vegetable juice ½ cup (125 ml)
Bok Choy, broccoli, collard, Chinese cabbage, 1 cup (250 ml) cooked
Kale, mustard greens or okra. Or 2 cups raw (500 ml)
Fortified tomato juice ½ cup (125 ml)

Fruits = 2 servings daily Serving size

Cut up or cooked fruit ½ cup (125ml)
Fruit juice ½ cup (125 ml)
Dried fruit ¼ cup (60 ml)
Calcium fortified fruit juice ½ cup (125 ml)
Figs 5

Fats = 3 to 6 servings daily
Oil, mayonnaise, soft margarine or ground flax seed 1 tsp (5ml)

Limit foods and beverages that are high in calories, fat, sugar or salt, such as desserts, fried snack foods, alcohol and sugar sweetened beverages.

Pay special attention to these nutrients when planning a vegetarian diet.

Protein: iron: vitamin B-12: calcium and vitamin D: omega-3 fats and zinc.

Protein plays an important role in the growth and repair of tissues in the body.it is made up of small units called amino acids; amino acids are the building blocks of your skin, muscle and organs.

Our bodies can make some of the amino acids that are needed to build protein, but others must come from the food we eat. These amino acids are called essential amino acids. Most plant sources of protein do not contain all the essential amino acids the body needs.

Eating a variety of vegetarian sources of protein throughout the day helps you to meet your protein needs.

Legumes are rich in protein and are also excellent sources of fibre, B-vitamins and iron. Legumes include kidney beans, soybeans, peas, lentils, black-eyed peas, chickpeas and lima beans.

To eat on their own or as a side dish, try soaking and cooking dried peas and beans before meal times or use canned legumes. Try legumes in recipes such as chili, baked beans, and soup and rice dishes.

Soy products are a good source of protein and can be great alternative for meat. They can boost the protein, calcium, and iron content of many dishes. Soy products can be used in just about any recipe.

Tofu or tempeh can be used in place of meat in many recipes. Tofu and tempeh are two different types of products made from soybeans. They can be crumbled, cubed, grilled, stir fried, or baked. Try marinating tofu or tempeh before cooking as they absorb flavors well.

Soy-based meat analogs (substitutes) such as veggie burgers, hot dogs and deli slices can be used in place of meat-based ones. Look for those that are fortified with extra minerals and vitamins such as vitamin B 12.

Fortified soy milk can be substituted for cow's milk in most recipes or enjoy it on its own.

Textured vegetable protein (TVP) is processed soybean protein that can look and taste like meat. TVP can be used in place of meat in recipes such as chili, tacos, sloppy joes, casseroles, or spaghetti sauce.

Soy flour will increase the protein content of baked products. A ½ cup supplies 22 grams of protein. Replace up to one half of the regular flour call for in your favorite recipes with soy flour.

Other vegetarian sources of protein include: milk and milk products, such as cheese, yogurt, eggs, nuts such as peanuts, almonds and cashews, seeds such as sunflower, pumpkin, and sesame, nut and seed butters, grain products such as quinoa, rice, breads, flours, pastas and cereals.

Iron: is a mineral that your body needs. Iron helps carry oxygen to all parts of your body and it helps form red blood cells. Women especially who are vegetarians, are at a greater risk of having low iron levels. Iron needs are increased for women aged 19 to 50 and during pregnancy. If the iron level in your body is low, you may feel weak, tired and look pale.

Iron that does not come from animal products is called non-heme iron.

Non-heme iron is found in vegetarian products such as:

Fortified breakfast cereals, tofu, pumpkin seeds, blackstrap molasses, legumes, such as beans, peas and lentils, baked potato with skin, almonds and cashews, almond and cashew butter, dried fruits such as apricots, currants, figs, prunes, raisins, greens such as broccoli, kale, bok Choy, soy based meat analogs such as vegetarian burgers, hot dogs, and deli slices.

Because non-heme iron is not absorbed as well as heme –iron from animal products, it is important to include a food source of vitamin C with your meals. Vitamin C helps your body absorb iron. Some sources of vitamin C include broccoli, green or red peppers, citrus fruit or juice, strawberries, tomatoes, and potatoes. If you drink tea or coffee, have it at least one hour before or after your meals. Tea and coffee contain compounds that can decrease your iron absorption. Calcium supplements can interfere with iron absorption. If you take calcium supplements, talk to your doctor about calcium and iron.

Vitamin B-12 plays a key role in maintaining the health of nerve cells and red blood cells. B-12 needs vary with stage of life: number of vitamin B 12 rich food servings needed each day; teens 13 years = 2 servings, teens 14 to 18 years = 3 servings, adults = 4 servings, pregnancy or breastfeeding = 4 servings.

B 12 is mainly found in animal products. However, there are a few plant based foods that have been fortified with vitamin B 12, fortified soy, rice or almond milk (½ cup) Cow's milk (½ cup) fortified breakfast cereals (1oz or 28 grams) soy based meat analogs such as veggie burgers, hot dogs or deli slices (1oz or 28 grams) you will need to check labels as not all labels as not all brands contain vitamin B-12; eggs (1 large) red star vegetarian support formula, nutritional yeast, (1 tbsp. or 3 grams) other brands are not reliable sources of vitamin B-12.

If you do not eat at least your recommended number of servings a day of vitamin B-12 rich foods, you will need to take a vitamin B-12 supplement of 5 to 10 mcg a day or 2,000 mcg a week. Talk to your doctor about vitamin B-12 supplement.

Calcium is a mineral that is important at all ages. Along with vitamin D, calcium helps to maintain healthy bones and to prevent osteoporosis.

These are foods that are sources of calcium: tofu processed with calcium (check labels) (½ cup = 1 serving), kale, broccoli, bok Choy = (1 cup cooked or 2 cups raw = 1 serving) cow's milk or yogurt (½ cup = 1 serving) cheese (¾oz or 21 grams = 1 serving) orange juice fortified with calcium (½ cup = 1 serving) calcium fortified soy, rice or almond milk (½ cup = 1 serving) calcium fortified breakfast cereal (1oz or 28 grams = 1 serving) almonds (1/4 cup = 1 serving) soybeans, cooked (½ cup = 1 serving) dried figs (5 = 1 serving).

Vitamin D works with calcium to help build strong bones and teeth. Your needs for vitamin D can be met by eating fortified foods, taking a vitamin D supplement, or from sunlight on your skin. The amount of vitamin D produced from sun on your skin depends on many factors including the strength of the sun where you live, time of year and your skin colour. Just a few minutes of sunlight on unprotected skin will increase your vitamin D, but for some people it may also increase the risk of sun damage.

What you need to eat to get enough vitamin D, cow's milk, breakfast cereal

(check labels) fortified soymilk and rice milk, margarine.

Omega – 3 fats are a type of fat that our bodies need. Omega -3 fats are important because of the role they play in normal growth and development. They are also important because they may play a role in preventing heart disease, high blood pressure, arthritis and cancer.

For non-vegetarians, fish is one of the best sources of omega-3 fats. However, there are other sources of omega -3 fats that can help to meet a vegetarian's needs. Include 2 servings of omega -3 fats every day in your diet. Pregnant and lactating women, as well as people with certain medical conditions, may need more in their diet.

Examples of one serving include: ground flaxseeds (1 tbsp.) or flaxseed oil

(1 tsp) canola or soybean oil, or margarine made with these oils (1 tbsp.) hemp seed oil (1tbsp.) and shelled hemp seeds (¼ cup) walnuts (¼ cup) soybeans, cooked (½ cup) and tofu (½ cup) omega – 3 eggs (1 each)

Zink is a nutrient that helps your immune system protect your body against disease, helps heal wounds, and is important for growth and development.

Getting enough zinc is important for vegetarians and non-vegetarians. Our bodies absorb less zinc from plant sources than from animal sources. Meeting your recommended number of daily servings from grains and legumes, nuts and other protein – rich foods will help you meet your daily zinc needs.

SAMPLE VEGETARIAN MENU

BREAKFAST = 1 cup oatmeal or 2 scrambled omega – 3 eggs
1 slice whole grain toast
1 to 2 tsp margarine
1 cup 1% milk or calcium fortified soy milk
1 banana

LUNCH = 1 cup vegetarian chili or baked beans
5 to 6 whole grain crackers
4 celery sticks
1 apple
1 cup 1% milk or calcium fortified soy milk

SNACK = 1 cup yogurt with 1 tsp ground flax seed
¼ cup tail mix

EVENING MEAL = 2 cups vegetarian stir fry with tofu
1 cup brown rice
1 cup fresh cantaloupe
1 cup calcium fortified orange juice

NIGHT SNACK = ¼ cup hummus
½ pita bread

EATING DISORDERS: are mental disorders defined by abnormal eating habits that negatively affect a person's physical or mental health. They include binge eating disorder where people eat a large amount of food in a short period of time.

Anorexia nervosa where people eat very little and have a low body weight: Bulimia nervosa where people eat a lot and then try to rid themselves of the food.

Pica where people eat non-food items, rumination disorder where people regurgitate food, avoidant / restrictive food intake disorder where people have a lack of interest in food, and a group of other specified feeding or eating disorders.

Anxiety disorder, depression, and substance abuse are common among people with eating disorders.

The cause of eating disorders is not clear, both biological and environmental factors appear to play a role. Cultural idealization of thinness is believed to contribute. Eating disorders affect about 12% of dancers.

Those who have experienced sexual abuse are also more likely to develop eating disorders.

Some disorders such as pica and rumination disorder occur more often in people with intellectual disabilities. Treatment can be effective for many eating disorders. This typically involves counselling, proper diet, and the reduction of efforts to eliminate food hospitalization is occasionally needed, medications may be used to help with some of the associated symptoms. At five years about 70% of people with anorexia and 50% of people with bulimia recover.

Recovery from binge eating disorder is less clear and estimated at 20% to 60%. Bothe anorexia and bulimia increase the risk of death.

Binge eating disorder affects about 1.6% of women and 0.8% of men in a given year. Anorexia affects about 0.4% and bulimia affects about 1.3% of young women in a given year.

Anorexia and bulimia occur nearly ten times more in females than males. Typically they begin in late childhood or early adulthood. Eating disorders appear to be lower in less developed countries.

Bulimia nervosa is a disorder characterized by binge eating and purging, as well as excessive evaluation of one's self-worth in terms of body weight or shape. Purging can include self-induced vomiting, over – exercising and the use of diuretics, enemas, and laxatives. Anorexia nervosa is characterized by extreme food restrictions and excessive weight loss, accompanied by the fear of being fat. The extreme weight loss often causes women and girls who have begun menstruating to stop having menstrual periods, a condition known as amenorrhea. The DSM-5 specifies two subtypes of anorexia nervosa, the restricting type and the binge / purge type.

Those who suffer from the restricting type of anorexia nervosa restrict food intake and do not engage in binge eating. However, those suffering from the binge/purge type lose control over their eating at least occasionally and may compensate for these binge episodes.

The most notable difference between anorexia nervosa binge/purge type and bulimia nervosa is the body weight of the person. Those diagnosed with anorexia nervosa binge/purge type are underweight, while those with bulimia nervosa may have a body weight that falls within the range from normal to obese. These eating disorders are specified as mental disorders in standard medical manuals.

Anorexia nervosa characterized by lack of maintenance of a healthy body weight, an obsessive fear of gaining weight or refusal to do so, and an unrealistic perception, or non- recognition of the seriousness, of current low body weight. Anorexia can cause menstruation to stop, and often leads to bone loss, loss of skin integrity, etc. it greatly stresses the heart, increasing the risk of heart attacks and related heart problems. The risk of death is greatly increased in individuals with this disease. The most underlining factor is it may not just be vanity, social, or media issue, but it could also be related to biological and or genetic components.

Bulimia nervosa characterized by recurrent binge eating followed by compensatory behaviors such as purging (self- induced vomiting, eating to the point of vomiting, excessive use of laxatives/ diuretics, or excessive exercise). Fasting and over- exercising may also be used as a method of purging following a binge. Muscle dysmorphia is characterized by appearance preoccupation that one's own is too small, too skinny, insufficiently muscular, or insufficiently lean. Muscle dysmorphia affects mostly males. Binge eating disorder, characterized by recurring binge eating at least once a week over a period of three months while experiencing lack of control, and guilt for overeating. The disorder can develop within individuals of a wide range of ages and socioeconomic classes.

Feeding or eating disorder is an eating or feeding disorder that does not meet full AN, or BN, criteria. Examples of otherwise- specified eating disorders include individuals with atypical anorexia nervosa, who meet all criteria for AN except being underweight, despite substantial weight loss; atypical bulimia nervosa, who meet all criteria for BN except that bulimic behaviors are less frequent or have not been ongoing for long enough, purging disorder, and night syndrome.

Compulsive overeating= individuals who habitually graze on large quantities of food rather than binging, as would be typical of binge eating disorder.

Diabulimia =characterized by the deliberate manipulation of insulin levels by diabetics in an effort to control their weight.

Food maintenance characterized by a set of aberrant eating behaviours of children in foster care.

Orthorexia nervosa, a term used to characterize an obsession with a pure diet, in which people develop an obsession with avoiding unhealthy foods to the point where it interferes with a person's life.

Selective eating disorder, also called picky eating, is an extreme sensitivity to how something tastes. A person with SED may or may not be a supertaster.

Drunkorexia, commonly characterized by purposely restricting food intake in order to reserve food calories for alcoholic calories exercising excessively in order to burn calories consumed from drinking.

Pregorexia, characterized by extreme dieting and over- exercising in order to control pregnancy weight gain: Under- nutrition during pregnancy is associated with low birth weight, coronary heart disease, type 2diabetes, stroke, hypertension, cardiovascular disease risk, and depression.

Symptoms and complications vary according to the nature and severity of the eating disorder.

Acne, xerosis, amenorrhoea, tooth loss, cavities, constipation, diarrhea, water retention and /or edema, lanugo, cardiac arrest, hypokalemia, death, osteoporosis, electrolyte imbalance, hyponatremia, brain atrophy, pellagra, scurvy, kidney failure, suicide.

Some physical symptoms of eating disorders are weakness, fatigue, sensitivity to cold, reduced beard growth in men, reduction in waking erections, reduced libido, weight loss and failure of growth. Unexplained hoarseness may be a symptom of an underlying eating disorder, as the result of acid reflux, or entry of acidic gastric material into the laryngoesophageal tract. Induced vomiting such as those with anorexia nervosa, binge eating, purging type or those with purging – type bulimia are at risk for acid reflux. Polycystic ovary syndrome is the most common endocrine disorder to affect women. Though often associated with obesity it can occur in normal weight individuals, it also is associated with binge eating and bulimic behavior.

The psychopathology of eating disorder centers around body image disturbance, such as concerns with weight and shape, self-worth being too dependent on weight and shape, fear of gaining weight even when underweight, denial of how severe the symptoms are and a distortion in the way the body is experienced.

Many people with eating disorders suffer from body dysmorphic disorder, altering the way a person sees himself or herself. A high proportion of individuals diagnosed with body dysmorphic disorder also had some type of eating disorder, with 15% of individuals having either anorexia or bulimia nervosa.

The link between body dysmorphic disorder and anorexia stems from the fact that both are characterized by a preoccupation with physical appearance and a distortion of body image. There are also many other possibilities such as interpersonal issues that could promote and sustain these illnesses. The media are oftentimes blamed for the incidence of eating disorders due to the fact that media images of idealized slim physical shape of people such as models and celebrities motivate or even force people to attempt to achieve slimness themselves.

The media are accused of distorting reality, in the sense that people portrayed are either naturally thin and are unrepresentative of normality, or unnaturally thin by forcing their bodies to look like the ideal image by putting excessive pressure on themselves to look a certain way. While past finding have described the cause of eating disorders as primarily psychological, environmental, and sociocultural, studies have uncovered evidence that there is a prevalent genetic/heritable aspect of the causes of eating disorders.

Personality traits there are various childhood personality traits associated with the development of eating disorders. During adolescence these traits may become intensified due to a variety of physiological and cultural influences such as the hormonal changes associated with puberty, stress related to the approaching demands of maturity and socio- cultural influences and perceived expectations, especially in areas that concern body image.

Eating disorders have been associated with a fragile sense of self and with disordered metallization. Many personality traits have a genetic component and are highly heritable. Maladaptive levels of certain traits may be acquired as a result of anoxic or traumatic brain injury, neurodegenerative diseases such as Parkinson's disease, neurotoxicity such as lead exposure, bacterial infection such as Lyme disease or viral infection, as well as hormonal influences.

People with gastrointestinal disorders= it has been documented that some people with celiac disease, irritable bowel syndrome or inflammatory bowel

Disease that are not conscious about the importance of strictly following their diet, choose to consume their trigger foods to promote weight loss. On the other hand, individuals with good dietary management may develop anxiety, food aversion and eating disorders because of concerns around cross contamination of their foods.

Child abuse which encompassed physical, psychological and sexual abuse, as well as neglect; has been shown by innumerable studies to be a precipitating factor in a wide variety of psychiatric disorders, including eating disorders. Children who are subjected to abuse may develop eating disorders in an effort to gain some sense of control or for a sense of comfort. They may be in an environment where the diet is unhealthy or insufficient.

Child abuse and neglect can cause profound changes in both the physiological structure and the neurochemistry of the developing brain. Children who, as wards of the state, were placed in orphanages or foster homes are especially susceptible to developing a disordered eating pattern.

A study in New Zealand 25% of the study subjects in foster care exhibited an eating disorder.

An unstable home environment is detrimental to the emotional well – being of children, even in the absence of blatant abuse or neglect the stress of an unstable home can contribute to the development of an eating disorder.

Social isolation has been shown to have a deleterious effect on an individual's physical and emotional well- being. Those that are socially isolated have a higher mortality rate in general as compared to individuals that have established social relationships. This effect on mortality is markedly increased in those with pre-existing medical or psychiatric conditions, and been especially noted in cases of coronary heart disease.

Social isolation can be inherently stressful, depressing and anxiety-provoking. In an attempt to ameliorate these distressful feelings an individual may engage in emotional eating in which food serves as a source of comfort.

The loneliness of social isolation and the inherent stressors associated have been implicated as triggering factors in binge eating.

Parental influence has been shown to be an intrinsic component in the development of eating behaviors of children. This influence is manifested and shaped by a variety of diverse factors such as familial genetic predisposition, dietary choices as dictated by cultural or ethnic preferences, the parents own body shape and eating patterns, the degree of involvement and expectations of their children's eating behavior as well as the interpersonal relationship of parent and child. This is in addition to the general psychosocial climate of the home and the presence or absence of a nurturing stable environment. It has been shown that maladaptive parental behavior has an important role in the development of eating disorders.

As to the more subtle aspects of parental influence, it has been shown that eating patterns are established in early childhood and that children should be allowed to decide when their appetite is satisfied as early as the age of two. A direct link has been shown between obesity and parental pressure to eat more. Coercive tactics in regard to diet have not been proven efficacious in controlling a child's eating behavior. Affection and attention have been shown to affect the degree of a child's acceptance of a more varied diet.

In the study of eating disorders, anorexia nervosa often occurs in girls who are high achievers, obedient, and always trying to please their parents. Their parents have a tendency to be over- controlling and fail to encourage the expression of emotions, inhibiting daughters from accepting their own feeling and desires.

Adolescent females in these overbearing families lack the ability to be independent from their families, yet realize the need to, often resulting in rebellion. Controlling their food intake may make them feel better, as it provides them with a sense of control.

In various studies, peer pressure was shown to be a significant contributor to body image concerns and attitudes towards eating in their teens and early twenties.

Teen girls concerns about their own weight, about how they appear to others and their perceptions that their peers want them to be thin are significantly related to weight –control behaviour. Another study showed that 40% of 9- and 10 year olds are already trying to lose weight. Such dieting is reported to be influenced by peer behavior.

Athletes have a significantly higher rate in eating disorders. Female athletes in sports such as gymnastics, ballet, diving, etc. are found to be at the highest risk among all athletes.

Women are more likely than men to acquire an eating disorder between the ages of 13-30. 0-15% of those with bulimia and anorexia are men.

There is a cultural emphasis on thinness which is especially pervasive in western society.

There is an unrealistic stereotype of what constitutes beauty and the ideal body type as portrayed by the media, fashion and entertainment industries. The cultural pressure on men and women to be perfect is an important predisposing factor for the development of eating disorders. Further, when women of all races base their evaluation of their self upon what is considered the culturally ideal body, the incidence of eating disorders increases.

Eating disorders are becoming more prevalent in non-western countries where thinness is not seen as the ideal, showing that social and cultural pressures are not the only causes of eating disorders.

Observations of anorexia in all of the non- western regions of the world point to the disorder not being culture-bound as once thought. Studies on rates of bulimia suggest that it might be culturally bound. In non- western countries, bulimia is less prevalent than anorexia, but these non- western countries where it is observed can be said to have probably or definitely been influenced or exposed to western culture and ideology.

Socioeconomic status has been viewed as a risk factor for eating disorders, presuming that possessing more resources allows for an individual to actively choose to diet and reduce body weight.

The media plays a major role in the way which people view themselves. Countless magazine ads and commercials depict thin celebrities like Lindsay Lohan, Nicole Richie, Victoria Beckham and Mary Kate Olsen, who appear to gain nothing but attention from their looks. Society has taught people that being accepted by others is necessary at all costs. Unfortunately this has led to the belief that in order to fit in on must look a certain way.

Athletes and eating disorders tend to go hand in hand, especially the sports where weight is a competitive factor; Gymnastics, horse- back riding, wrestling, body building, and dancing fall into this category of weight dependent sports.

Eating disorders especially women, that participate in competitive activities, often lead to having physical and biological changes related to their weight that often mimic prepubescent stages.

Often as women's bodies change they lose their competitive edge which leads them to take extreme measures to maintain their younger body shape.

Men often struggle with binge eating followed by excessive exercise while focusing on building muscle rather than losing fat, this goal of gaining muscle is just as much an eating disorder as obsessing over thinness.

The estimated percentage of athletes that struggle with eating disorders based in the category of sport=dance, figure skating, gymnastics- 35% Judo and wrestling = 29% cycling, swimming, running = 20% golf, high jumping= 14% volleyball, soccer = 12% although most of these athletes develop eating disorders to keep their competitive edge, others use exercise as a way to maintain their weight and figure. This is just as regulating food intake for competition. Even though there is mixed evidence showing at what point athletes are challenged with eating disorders, studies show that regardless of competition level all athletes are at a higher risk for developing eating disorders than non-athletes; especially those that participate in sports where thinness is a factor.

Pressure from society is also seen within the homosexual community. Homosexual men are at greater risk of eating disorder symptoms than heterosexual men. Within the gay culture, muscularity gives the advantages of both social and sexual desirability and also power. These pressures and ideas that another homosexual male may desire a mate who is thinner or muscular can possibly lead to eating disorders.

While there are many influences to how an individual processes their body image, the media does play a major role. Parental and peer influence, and self –efficacy beliefs also play a large role in an individual's view of themselves.

The way the media presents images can have a lasting effect on an individual's perception of their body image. Eating disorders are a world-wide issue and while women are more likely to be affected by an eating disorder it still affects both genders. The media has an impact on eating disorders whether shown in a positive or negative light, it then has a responsibility to use caution when promoting images that project an ideal that many turn to eating disorders to attain.

Biochemical: eating behavior is a complex process controlled by the neuroendocrine system, of which the hypothalamus- pituitary – adrenal-axis is a major component.

Dysregulation of the HPA axis has been associated with eating disorders, such as irregularities in the manufacture, amount or transmission of certain neurotransmitters, hormones or neuropeptides and amino acids such as homocysteine, elevated levels of which are found in AN and BN as well as depression.

Serotonin: a neurotransmitter involved in depression also has an inhibitory effect on eating behaviour.

Norepinephrine is both a neurotransmitter and a hormone; abnormalities in either capacity may affect eating behaviour.

Dopamine: in addition to being a precursor of norepinephrine is also a neurotransmitter which regulates the rewarding property of food.

Neuropeptide Y also known as NPY is a hormone that encourages eating and decreases metabolic rate. Blood levels of NPY are elevated in patients with anorexia nervosa, and have shown that injection of this hormone into the brain of rats with restricted food intake increases their time spent running on a wheel. Normally the hormone stimulates eating in healthy patients, but under conditions of starvation it increases their activity rate, probably to increase the chance of finding food. The increase of NPY in the blood of patients with eating disorders can in some ways explain the instances of extreme over-exercising found in anorexia nervosa patients.

Leptin and ghrelin: is a hormone produced primarily by the fat cells in the body; it has an inhibitory effect on appetite by inducing a feeling of satiety.

Ghrelin is an appetite inducing hormone produced in the stomach and the upper portion of the small intestine. Circulating levels of both hormones are an important factor in weight control. While often associated with obesity, both hormones and their respective effects have been implicated in the pathophysiology of anorexia nervosa and bulimia nervosa.

Leptin can also be used to distinguish between constitutional thinness found in a healthy person with a low BMI and an individual with anorexia nervosa.

Gut bacteria and immune system: studies have shown that a majority of patients with anorexia and bulimia nervosa have elevated levels of autoantibodies that affect hormones and neuropeptides that regulate appetite control and the stress response. Lesions to the right frontal lobe or temporal lobe can cause pathological symptoms of an eating disorder.

Tumors in various regions of the brain have been implicated in the development of abnormal eating patterns. Brain calcification a study highlights a case in which prior calcification of the right thalamus; may have contributed to development of anorexia nervosa.

Somatosensory homunculus is the representation of the body located in the somatosensory cortex. The illustration was originally termed Penfield's Homunculus meaning little man. In normal development this representation should adapt as the body goes through its pubertal growth spurt. However, in AN, it is hypothesized that there is a lack of plasticity in this area, which may result in impairments of sensory processing and distortion of body image. Obstetric complications: studies done show maternal smoking, obstetric and perinatal complications such as maternal anemia, very pre-term birth (less than 32 weeks), being born small for gestational age, neonatal cardiac problems, preeclampsia, placental infraction at birth increase the risk factor for developing either anorexia or bulimia nervosa.

The initial diagnosis should be made by a competent medical professional. The medical history is the most powerful tool for diagnosing eating disorders. There are many medical disorders that mimic eating disorders and comorbid psychiatric disorders.

All organic causes should be ruled out prior to a diagnosis of an eating disorder or any other psychiatric disorder.

In the past 30 years eating disorders have become increasingly conspicuous and it is uncertain whether the changes in presentation reflect a true increase. Anorexia nervosa and bulimia nervosa are the most clearly defined subgroups of a wider range of eating disorders.

The diagnostic workup typically includes complete medical and psychosocial history and follows a rational and formulaic approach to the diagnosis. Neuroimaging using MRI and PET scans have been used to detect cases in which a lesion, tumor or other organic condition has been either the sole causative or contributory factor in an eating disorder.

There are multiple medical conditions which may be misdiagnosed as primary psychiatric disorder, complicating or delaying treatment. These may have a synergistic effect in conditions which mimic an eating disorder or on a properly diagnosed eating disorder.

Lyme disease: which is known as the great imitator, as it may present a variety of psychiatric or neurological disorders including anorexia nervosa. Gastrointestinal disease such as celiac disease, peptic ulcer, eosinophilic esophagitis or non- celiac gluten sensitivity, celiac disease is also known as the great imitator, because it may involve several organs and cause an extensive variety of non-gastrointestinal symptoms, such as psychiatric and neurological disorders, including anorexia nervosa.

Addison's disease is a disorder of the adrenal cortex which in decreased hormonal production. Addison's disease, even in subclinical form may mimic many of the symptoms of anorexia nervosa.

Gastric adenocarcinoma is one of the most common forms of cancer in the world. Complications due to this condition have been misdiagnosed as an eating disorder.

Psychological disorders which could be confused with an eating disorder.

Emetophobia is an anxiety disorder characterized by an intense fear of vomiting. A person so afflicted may develop rigorous standards of food hygiene, such as not touching food with their hands. They may become socially withdrawn to avoid situations which in their perception may make them vomit. Many who suffer from emetophobia are diagnosed with anorexia or self-starvation. In severe cases of emetophobia they may drastically reduce their food intake.

Phagophobia is an anxiety disorder characterized by a fear of eating; it is usually initiated by an adverse experience while eating such as choking or vomiting. A person with this disorder may complain of pain while swallowing.

Body dysmorphic disorder (BDD) is listed as a somatoform disorder that affects up to 2% of the population. It is characterized by excessive rumination over and actual or perceived physical flaw. BDD has been diagnosed equally among men and women. BDD has been misdiagnosed as anorexia nervosa, it also occurs in 39% if eating disorder cases. BDD is a chronic and debilitating condition which may lead to social isolation, major depression and suicidal ideation and attempts.

Prevention aims to promote a healthy development before the occurrence of eating disorders. It also intends early identification of an eating disorder before it is too late to treat. Children as young as 5-7 are aware of the cultural messages regarding body image and dieting, prevention comes in bringing these issues to the light, discuss the following with your children.

Emotional bites: a simple way to discuss emotional eating is to ask children about why they might eat besides being hungry, talk about more effective ways to cope with emotions, emphasizing the value of sharing feelings with you.

Say no to teasing: emphasize that it is wrong to say hurtful things about other people's body size.

Body talk: the importance of listening to one's body, eating when you are hungry (not starving), and stop when you are satisfied (not stuffed) children intuitively grasp these concepts.

Fitness: educate your children about the genetics of body size and the normal changes occurring in the body, and discuss their hopes and fears on growing bigger. Focus on fitness and a balanced diet.

Treatment varies according to type and severity of eating disorder, treatment can take place in a variety of settings, community programs, hospitals, day programs, and group.

Cognitive behavioral therapy, which postulates that an individual's feelings and behaviors are caused by their own thoughts instead of external stimuli such as other people, situations or events; the idea is to change how a person thinks and reacts to a situation even if the situation itself does not change.

Treatment can be expensive due to limitations in health care coverage; people hospitalized with anorexia nervosa may be discharged while still underweight, resulting in relapse and re-hospitalisation. For children with anorexia, the only well- established treatment is the family treatment behaviour.

Outcomes estimates are complicated by non-uniform criteria used by various studies, but for anorexia nervosa, bulimia nervosa, and binge eating disorder, 85% range, with larger proportions of people experiencing at least partial remission. Outcome of eating disorders vary, for many it can be a lifelong struggle or it can be overcome within months, in the United States, twenty million women and ten million men have an eating disorder, at least once in their lifetime. Depending on the type of eating disorder, the age it began, previous psychiatric disorders etc., the severity of the outcome differs.

Pregnant women with a binge eating disorder have shown to have a greater chance of having a miscarriage compared to pregnant women with any other eating disorder.

An individual who is in remission is at a high risk of falling back into the habit of self- harming themselves factors such as high stress regarding their job, pressures from society, as well as other occurrences that inflict stress on a person, can push a person back to what they feel will ease the pain.

People who are showing signs of attachment anxiety will most likely have trouble communicating their emotional status as well as having trouble seeking effective social support.

Signs that a person has adopted this symptom include not showing recognition to their caregiver when he /she are feeling pain. More severe eating disorder symptoms directly correspond to higher attachment anxiety. The more this symptom increases, the more difficult it is to achieve eating disorder reduction prior to treatment.

Anorexia nervosa symptoms include the increasing chance of getting osteoporosis. This disease causes the bones of an individual to become brittle, weak, and low in density. Thinning of the hair as well as dry hair and skin is also very common. The muscles of the heart will also start to change if no treatment is inflicted on the person. This causes the heart to have abnormally slow heart rate along with low blood pressure. Heart failure becomes a major consideration when this begins to occur. Muscles throughout the body begin to lose their strength. This will cause the individual to begin feeling faint, drowsy, and weak. The body will begin to grow a layer of hair called lanugo. The human body does this in response to the lack of heat and insulation due to the low percentage of body fat.

Bulimia nervosa symptoms include heart problems like an irregular heartbeat that can lead to heart failure and death. This occurs because of the electrolyte imbalance that is a result of the constant binge and purge process.

The probability of a gastric rupture increases; a gastric rupture is when there is a sudden rupture of the stomach lining that can be fatal. The acids that are contained in the vomit can cause a rupture in the esophagus as well as tooth decay. As a result, to laxative abuse, irregular bowel movements may occur along with constipation. Sores along the lining of the stomach called peptic ulcers begin to appear and the chance of developing pancreatitis increases.

Binge eating symptoms include high blood pressure, which can lead to heart disease if not treated, an increase in the levels of cholesterol, the chance of being diagnosed with gallbladder disease increases, which affects the digestive tract.

Eating disorders result in about 7,000 deaths a year, making them the mental illness with the highest mortality rate

Eating disorders are illnesses that affect all aspects of a child's or adolescent's life. Anorexia nervosa is one type of eating disorder that is very difficult for many people to understand. Anorexia nervosa is a serious, potentially life- threating disorder characterized by self- starvation and excessive weight loss.

This disorder often begins during adolescence, frequently around the time of puberty. Children and adolescence with anorexia nervosa have an overwhelming fear of being overweight, and an extreme drive to be thin. This will lead them to behaviors that will cause weight loss, including cutting back on becomes obsessed with food and dieting. They may also become dangerously thin. No matter how thin they get, they think they are still fat or they may then be terrified of becoming fat; some will exercise excessively to burn off the calories. They may count calories or grams of fat, starve themselves, limit types of food they allow themselves to eat, purging or vomiting their food (otherwise known as anorexia bulimia sub type), taking laxatives, diet pills, avoiding to eat in front of people and making excuses like "I'm not hungry" "my stomach hurts" or "I don't have time to".

Eating disorder facts: at least 1 in 10 people who develop eating disorders are boys. Most children or adolescents get help for an eating disorder because their parents insist they get help; not because they want to get help.

20% of patients with eating disorders will die of their illness. With treatment,

About 75% to 80% of adolescents with an eating disorder will recover.

We were all made differently. There are many possible combinations of shapes and sizes that compose a person's body. It is possible for someone to naturally be dense boned. Just as likely as it is for someone to be naturally model thin. Someone could be eating a balanced diet, exercising moderately and still be fat, but they can still be healthy as well.

Symptoms and results of anorexia nervosa:

Yellow – orange tinged skin, thinning of the hair or hair that breaks easily, growth of downy hair on back, stomach, or the side of the face,

Major weight loss in a short period of time, failure to gain weight or height normally, delay on onset of puberty, loss of menstrual periods, low body temperature, counting calories and fat, dieting, food rules, eating alone, increasing interest in all things to do with food, disgust for previously favorite foods, frequent weighing, wearing baggy clothes, distorted body image, excessive exercise, extreme concern with appearance, and so much more.

Recovery: I like to think that eating and discussions are the cure to anorexia. Food is our medicine. If someone were to just discuss about their problems, but not eat, these eating disorder thoughts would stay with them and everything discussed would go in one ear and out the other. It is just not possible to recover without eating. Our bodies need glucose, without it our brains go a little funky and we can't think straight. We don't think rationally. Without having a clear mind and being able to think things through; we would still be occupied with the same old thoughts of food, losing weight, and not trying to get fat. The healthier your weight becomes the less chance of relapsing or lapsing.

How much food do I need: Everybody is different and we all need different amounts? For example: an average 13 year old would probably consume between 1600 and 2500 calories a day. It depends on age, height, gender, activity level and genes. So when an anorexia child loses a vast quantity of weight, it is expected for them to gain it back. But the amount of food needed, varies according to how far along they are with their eating disorder. Someone who is at the point of death knocking at their door would probably need a minimum of 3000 calories, probably around 5000 to 6000 or so a day. But if you suddenly start feeding someone who has been starving themselves for a while, their body can go into shock, there can be electrolyte imbalances, extreme bloating and constipation, vomiting and the body rejecting food and heart attack; which can all lead to death.

This is why it is so important to start of slowly and work your way up. I would say start off with about 800 calories a day and every 2-3 days add an extra 100-300 calories a day until you reach around 2000. From there you can determine whether you need to increase or continue with 2000. While re-feeding it is important that the anorexic person does not exercise. You cannot afford for them to lose more weight.

Here are some meal plans with different amounts of calories

The starter plan= 800 calories:

Breakfast: ½ cup oat meal cooked in water

Snack: an ensure regular or plus calories or a fruit smoothie

Lunch: a bowl of rice with chicken or some other form of protein such as beans,

Ham or beef

Snack: ensure regular or fruit smoothie

Dinner: ½ cup rice, a small amount of chicken and some steamed vegetables.

Or a bowl of vegetable based soup

Once the body is ready to move onto solids you can move on to this plan

Next step = 1200 calories

Breakfast: 1 slice of bread with one tbsp. peanut butter and jam

Snack: ensure plus calories

Lunch: ½ ham and cheese sandwich

Snack: ½ of a 6 inch tortilla with hummus and grated carrots

Dinner: ½ cup of rice with 3oz chicken, steamed vegetables, and 8oz whole milk

Or spaghetti and meatballs with a side Caesar salad and 8oz whole milk

Snack: ensure plus or fruit smoothie

Once you become more comfortable eating a variety of foods and larger quantities.

Accepting naughty foods= 1800 calories

Breakfast: 2 slices of bread with butter, one egg and juice or a fruit salad

Or 1 cup oatmeal cooked with vanilla ensure and ¼ cup raisins

Snack: something you love, but would never let your-self eat e.g. cookies and milk, ice cream and fruit, cheese and crackers.

Lunch: a ham, chicken, tuna meat, egg or turkey sandwich with either carrot sticks and an apple or a juice box

Snack: another small quantity of naughty food and milk, but be sure to include some nutritious foods like fruit and dairy

Dinner: 1 cup rice, ½ large chicken breast, ½ cup steamed veggies, a side salad and 8oz whole milk

Snack: green smoothie or fruit juice (something light)

When your body adjusts to this amount of foods

You can step it up a notch to= 2500 calories

Breakfast: 2/3 cup yogurt, ½ cup of granola, ½ cup of fruit

Snack: granola bar and fruit smoothie

Lunch: large bagel with 2-4 tbsp. peanut butter and banana, cookies and milk

Snack: veggies and hummus

Dinner: whole wheat pasta with tomato sauce and chicken, meat sauce or cheese sauce, a side salad with dressing, a slice garlic bread and a glass of whole milk (you can also substitute with any other milk alternative)

Snack: cereal and milk or fruit and nuts

You will be on the right track getting to where you want to be when you are eating 3000 - 3500 calories

Breakfast: 1 cup granola, 6oz yogurt and ¾ cup fruit

Snack: energy bar and milk

Lunch: 2 slices of homemade or store bought vegetable pizza with a side of carrot sticks and fruit

Snack: ensure plus and a muffin

Dinner: baked sweet potato, chicken, steamed vegetables and salad with dressing

Snack: dessert of your choice and glass of milk

(This is a very complicated confusing and deadly disease I hope those of you looking for information on this subject now know more about what you are dealing with)

Start talking with your children and family; to me prevention is worth a pound of cure (meaning if you can prevent it you should) be more involved. Start listening; instead of talking you never know you just might learn something.

Good luck and God bless you.

Nutrition and recovery from Anorexia Nervosa

Recovering from the malnutrition (underweight and growth delay) experienced in anorexia nervosa is hard work:

People experiencing malnutrition & in the early stages of nutrition rehabilitation can become medically unwell and should see their doctor regularly. (Your doctor will manage any electrolyte or body salt problems medically).

Food is the medicine for recovery from malnutrition. To fully recover (i.e. to recover weight and restart normal growth) you need to build up to eating more than most people might expect and enjoy, for some weeks and months.

Being in a malnourished or starved state causes a number of symptoms that may make it hard to accomplish meals easily: feeling full quickly and for a prolonged time, suppressed appetite, being more worried, anxious and indecisive, and feeling that you can't stop thinking about food. In eating disorders people have become worried about how much food to eat and fearful about their weight.

The aim of nutrition in recovery is to supply sufficient energy (from protein, carbohydrates and fats) foods to rebuild lost tissue. Any insufficiencies in vitamins and minerals intake must be replaced. Generally increasing food intake will replace most of the micronutrient deficits, but some may require additional iron, zinc or calcium. A multi vitamin and mineral supplement (at the recommended dietary intake dosage) may be useful.

Everyday family foods are recommended, most people need to re-introduce more bread and cereal foods, more milk and milk products, more meat and protein rich foods, more healthy fat rich foods. No specialized foods are required. However, foods like ensure may be helpful if you are having trouble eating enough.

Initially an underweight\ malnourished person will have lower than expected food needs and will restore weight and health by building up to an intake of 1500 – 2000 calories daily; aiming for a weight gain rate of 500g \per week.

Within a few weeks most people will find they require more than this and will need to increase their intake to around 3000 calories or more in order to fully recover and return to full physical health.

This translates into a plan of meals providing; 3 regular meals + 3 regular snacks it is important to remember that weight may appear to increase quickly for the first week or two. This is mostly due to improved hydration, as people experiencing malnutrition are usually dehydrated. It is recommended that you work closely with a doctor and dietitian at this time.

Weight gain is a sensitive subject as anyone skinny enough to be contemplating weight gain is eyed with suspicion and envy especially among women in whom thinness is particularly celebrated. With only 2% of the population underweight and a staggering two thirds (66%) overweight, it is easy (though not right) to see why there is little support. However, while obesity is often the result of poor lifestyle choices, underweight is mostly due to genetics and little to do with poor decision making. Unfortunately, rather than getting a little empathy, as after all it is out of your control, there is often little understanding or support for those who desire to gain weight.

Being underweight is defined as having a body mass index (BMI) BELOW 18.5. This is estimated to be less than the body mass needed to sustain optimal health. Conversely, over 25 is considered overweight and over 30 is considered obese.

However keep in mind that there are many problems with the BMI scale, which only looks at weight and height it does not take muscle into account.

Some people are naturally very skinny but still healthy. Being underweight according to this scale does not necessarily mean that you have a health problem. Obesity is currently one of the world's biggest health problems.

However, being underweight may be just as bad for your health as being obese.

According to one study, being underweight was associated with a 140% greater risk of early death in men and 100% in women.

In this study, obesity was only associated with a 50% greater risk of early death, indicating that being underweight may be even worse for your health.

Being underweight can also impair immune function, raise your risk of infections, and lead to osteoporosis and fractures, and cause fertility problems.

People who are underweight are also much more likely to get sarcopenia (age related muscle wasting), and may be at greater risk of dementia.

Bottom line: Being underweight can be just as unhealthy as being obese, if not more. People who are underweight are at risk of osteoporosis, infections, fertility problems and early death.

Several things can cause someone to become underweight.

Eating disorders: this includes anorexia nervosa, a serious mental disorder.

Thyroid problems; having an overactive thyroid (hyperthyroidism) can boost metabolism and cause unhealthy weight loss.

Celiac disease: the most severe form of gluten intolerance. Most people with celiac disease don't know that they have it.

Diabetes: having uncontrolled diabetes (mainly type 1) can lead to severe weight loss.

Cancer: cancerous tumors often burn large amount of calories and can cause someone to lose a lot of weight.

Infections: certain infections can cause someone to become severely underweight. This includes parasites, tuberculosis and HIV/ AIDS.

If you are underweight, then you may want to see your doctor in order to rule out a serious medical condition. This is particularly important if you have recently started losing large amounts of weight without even trying.

Bringing on soda and donuts may help you gain weight, but it can destroy your health at the same time.

If you are underweight then you want to gain a balanced amount of muscle mass and subcutaneous fat, not a bunch of unhealthy belly fat.

There are plenty of normal weight people who get type 2diabetes, heart disease and other health problems often associated with obesity.

It is absolutely essential that you still eat healthy foods and live an overall healthy lifestyle.it is very important to eat mostly healthy foods even if you are trying to gain weight.

Eat more than your body burns: The most important thing you can do to gain weight is to eat more calories than your body needs.

If you want to gain weight slowly and steadily, then aim for 300-500 calories more than you burn each day. If you want to gain weight fast, then aim for something like 700-1000 calories above your maintenance level.

You will not need to count calories for the rest of your life, but it helps to do it for the first few weeks to get a feel for how many calories you are eating daily.

Eat lots of protein: the single most important nutrient for gaining healthy weight is protein.

Muscle is made of protein, and without it most of those extra calories may end up as body fat. However, keep in mind that protein is a double-edged sword. It is also highly filling, so that can reduce your hunger and appetite significantly. This can make it harder to get in enough calories.

High – protein foods include meats, fish, eggs, many dairy products, legumes, nuts and others. Protein forms the building blocks of your muscles. Eating sufficient protein is required to gain muscle weight instead of just fat.

Eat plenty of high-carb and high-fat foods if weight gain is a priority for you. It is best to eat plenty of protein, fat and carbs at each meal.

Make sure to eat at least 3 meals per day, and try to add in energy – dense snacks whenever possible.

Eat a lot of energy dense foods and use sauces, spices and condiments.

It is very important to eat mostly whole, single ingredient foods. Using plenty of spices, sauces and condiments can help. The tastier your food is, the easier it is to eat a lot of it. Try to emphasize energy dense foods as much as possible. These are foods that contain many calories relative to their weight.

Like: almonds, walnuts, macadamia nuts, peanuts, raisins, dates, prunes and others, whole milk, full- fat yogurt, cheese, and cream.

Grains whole grains like oats and brown rice.

Meats: chicken, beef, lamb, pork. Choose fattier cuts.

Potatoes: sweet potatoes and yams. Dark chocolate, avocados, peanut butter, coconut milk, granola and trail mixes.

Many of these foods are very filling, and sometimes you may need to force yourself to keep eating even if you feel full.

Eating whole fruit is fine, but; try to emphasize fruit that doesn't require too much chewing like bananas

It is important to lift heavy weights to improve your strength. This will help you gain muscle mass instead of just fat.

Combining a high calorie intake with heavy strength training are the two most important factors. Here are some tips to help you to gain weight faster

Do not drink water before meals as this can fill your stomach and make it harder to get in enough calories.

Eat more often: squeeze in additional meals or snacks whenever you can; Such as before bed.

Drink milk; drink whole milk to quench it and add calories.

Use bigger plates if you are trying to get in more calories, as smaller cause people to automatically eat less.

Add cream to your coffee.

Get enough sleep; sleeping properly is very important for muscle growth.

Eat your protein first and vegetables last; if you have a mix of foods on your plate, eat the calorie – dense and protein rich foods first. Eat the vegetables last.

Your body has a certain set point of weight where it feels comfortable. Whether you are trying to lose or gain weight your body resists changes.

When you eat more calories and gain weight, you can expect your body to respond by reducing your appetite and boosting your metabolism. This is largely mediated by the brain, as well as weight regulating hormones like leptin.

So you should expect a certain level of difficulty, in some cases, you may literally need to force yourself to eat despite feeling full.

At the end of the day, changing your weight is a marathon, not a sprint. It can take a long time, and you need to be consistent in order to succeed.

If you are underweight or simply trying to gain more weight, then the following high calorie meal plans will help you to reach your goal.

They are designed to help you gain weight in a healthy way.

Ok let's get started

Day 1 – 2896 calories

Breakfast = ½ cup granola, 3.5oz Greek yogurt, 4oz orange juice

Toppings 1oz chopped Brazil nuts, ¼ cup each blueberries & raspberries

Total calories breakfast =700

Morning snack = 2 oatcakes (oat crackers), 1 tbsp. peanut butter, 1 nectarine

Total calories = 246

Lunch = 1 whole wheat pita bread, 4oz roast chicken,

1 med avocado, sliced or mashed, large handful of spinach and

Watercress and 8oz 3% milk

Total calories = 700

Afternoon snack = 2oz trail mix

Total calories = 250

Dinner = 5oz salmon fillet, 3.5oz brown basmati rice (dry weight)

3oz cooked broccoli, tossed in 1 tbsp. tahini and a squeeze of lemon

3oz green peas

Total calories = 900

Evening snack = medium banana

Total calories = 100

I know this looks like a lot of food, however, try to eat as much as you can and work it up until this is comfortable for you without feeling stuffed. It will probably take a week or two take your time slow gets the job done.

Day two calories = 3001

Breakfast = scrambled eggs on rye toast (3 eggs and two slices of rye buttered toast) ½ cup prune juice

Total calories = 671

Morning snack = 1oz pumpkin seeds, 1 pear

Total calories = 226

Lunch = quinoa & mozzarella salad

3.5oz quinoa, cooked, 2oz mozzarella, 1oz toasted pine nuts

1 large handful of baby spinach, 1 tbsp. olive oil, 1 bunch fresh basil

Total calories = 819

Afternoon snack = 3 oat cakes (oat crackers), 3 tbsp. hummus

Total calories = 233

Dinner = shrimp (prawn) & cherry tomato pasta

5oz whole wheat spelt penne, 4oz shrimp, 3oz cherry tomatoes,

1 tbsp. olive oil, 2 tbsp. chopped parsley

Salad = 2 cups mixed salad, 1 tbsp. olive oil, 1 tsp balsamic vinegar

Total calories = 750

Evening snack = blend ½ banana, 1 tbsp. almond butter, ½ cup blueberries,

5oz whole milk yogurt

Total calories = 302

Day 3 calories = 2996

Breakfast = blueberry, nut and cinnamon oatmeal

2oz oats, 1 cup whole milk, 1oz raisins, 2 tbsp. ground almonds,

½ tsp cinnamon, topping, 1oz walnuts or pecans, ¼ cup blueberries

½ cup grape juice

Total calories = 821

Morning snack = large handful cashew nuts and raisins

Total calories = 185

Lunch = 3.5oz smoked mackerel fillet, mashed with 2 tbsp. natural yogurt,

1 tbsp. chopped dill, a squeeze of lemon and black pepper

6 oat cakes (oat crackers), 1 apple

Total calories = 778

Afternoon snack = granola bar

Total calories = 119

Dinner = 4oz grilled steak fillet, baked potato with garlic butter, spinach and

Green beans, sautéed I 1 tbsp. olive oil

Total calories = 760

Evening snack = 6oz Greek yogurt, small banana sliced, 4oz crushed walnuts

And 4oz crushed dark chocolate

Total calories = 333

Day 4 calories = 3357

Vegetarian meal plan for weight gain

Breakfast = 3 vegetarian sausages, 2 grilled portabella mushrooms,

1 large grilled tomato, 3oz baked beans, 2 slices buttered whole

Wheat toast, 1 cup pineapple juice

Total calories = 728

Morning snack = blend 1 small banana, 1 tbsp. almond butter, 3.5oz Greek

Yogurt, 1tsp honey, water too thin as necessary

Total calories = 288

Lunch = goats cheese, walnut & cranberry salad

2oz goat's cheese, 3oz mixed salad leaves, 2oz cherry tomatoes,

1oz walnuts, 2 tbsp. dried cranberries, 1 tbsp. olive oil,

1 tbsp. balsamic vinegar and 2 whole wheat pita breads

Total calories = 835

Afternoon snack = 2 rye crackers, 2 tbsp. cream cheese, 1oz pumpkin seeds

Total calories = 337

Dinner = zucchini and parmesan frittata
3 eggs, 1 zucchini, (sautéed), 2oz parmesan, 1 tbsp. olive oil for cooking
1 medium sweet potato, cut into wedges, roasted in 1 tbsp. sunflower
Oil, green salad, dressed with 1 tbsp. olive oil and lemon juice
Total calories = 957
Evening snack = 4oz dark chocolate total calories = 212
Day 5 total calories = 3146
Vegan meal plan for weight gain
Breakfast = 2 slices whole wheat toast, 3 tbsp. peanut butter,
Large bowl fruit salad
Total calories = 789
Morning snack = oatmeal raisin bar
Total calories = 240
Lunch = lentil & avocado salad
3 cups spinach and watercress salad, ½ avocado, cubed, ½ cup cooked
Brown and green lentils, 1oz toasted pine nuts,
Dressing 1 tbsp. olive oil, squeeze of lemon juice
Total calories = 565
Afternoon snack = 10 Brazil nuts, 1 banana
Total calories = 245

Dinner = 3.5oz soba noodles (dry weight), 3.5oz firm tofu, 2oz cashew nuts,
1 tbsp. sesame oil, ½ cup broccoli, ½ cup baby corn
Total calories = 955
Evening snack = 1/3 tub hummus, carrot and celery sticks,
Total calories = 352

Each meal should contain 750 calories, and each snack 250 calories.

Include as many food groups such as: fruits, vegetables, grains, protein food and dairy as possible at each meal and snack to ensure that you meet your daily vitamin and mineral needs.

Sample of high calorie breakfast
1 cup oatmeal made with 2 cups of whole milk
Top it with 12 sliced almonds and ¼ cup of raisins

1 cup orange juice

Total calories = 730

Or

Veggie omelet = 3 eggs, ½ cup sliced mushrooms, 1oz Swiss cheese,

1 tsp vegetable oil, 2 slices of whole wheat bread toasted with 1 tsp butter,

1 cup whole milk.

Total calories =750

Sample high calorie lunch

½ cup hummus, 1.5oz feta cheese, alfalfa sprouts, and shredded carrots,

Stuffed into a whole-wheat pita, 5oz Greek yogurt, large banana

Total calories = 740

Or

Two slices cheese pizza, 2 cups salad greens topped with 2 tbsp. salad dressing

Total calories = 760

Sample high calorie dinner

4oz grilled salmon, drizzled with 1 tsp olive oil, 1 cup brown rice, 1 cup peas,

1 ½ cups fresh pineapple

Total calories = 745

Or

Burger made with 4oz lean hamburger meat, on whole wheat bun,

1 ½ cups roasted red potatoes, made with 2 tsp olive oil,

1 ½ cups roasted cauliflower drizzled with 1 tsp olive oil

Total calories = 750

Snacks for in-between meals and before bed

Snack calories should = 250

Examples would be = large apple with 2 tbsp. peanut butter.

Or

Turkey sandwich made with 1oz turkey, one eighth avocado on one slice whole wheat bread.

Or

1 cup of unsweetened cereal with 1 cup whole milk

While the concept of weight gain is really simple, actually making it happen and happen properly is hard for many people, however, all it takes is three simple steps.

Eat enough calories

Get the rest of your diet right (protein, fat, carbs, etc.).

That's all it takes, in most cases you should eat 300-500 additional calories per day. If your calorie intake is accurate, you should gain 0.5 to 1 pound per week.

Weigh yourself once a week (always first thing in the morning on an empty stomach) to make sure weight gain is taking place as fast as it should be. If it is then you are perfect. If you are gaining weight slower, you need to add an additional 300 calories daily to your diet.

Whenever you end up gaining weight in that ideal range per week you are perfect. Keep eating that amount of calories.

HYPOTHYROIDISM (UNDERACTIVE THYRIOD)

Hypothyroidism is a condition in which your thyroid gland doesn't produce enough of certain important hormones.

Women, especially those older than age 60, are more likely to have hypothyroidism; it upsets the normal balance of chemical reactions in your body. It seldom causes symptoms in the early stages, but over time, untreated hypothyroidism can cause a number of health problems, such as obesity, joint pain, infertility and heart disease.

The good news is that accurate thyroid tests are available to diagnose hypothyroidism with synthetic thyroid hormone is usually simple, safe, and effective once you and your doctor find the right dose for you.

Symptoms and causes

The signs and symptoms of hypothyroidism vary, depending on the severity of the hormone deficiency. But in general, any problems you have tend to develop slowly over a number of years. At first you may barely notice the symptoms of hypothyroidism, such as fatigue and weight gain, or you may simply attribute them to getting older. But as your metabolism, continues to slow, you may develop more- obvious signs and symptoms. Hypothyroidism signs and symptoms may include: fatigue, increased sensitivity to cold, constipation, dry skin, weight gain, puffy face, hoarseness, muscle weakness, elevated blood cholesterol level, muscle aches, tenderness and stiffness, pain, stiffness, or swelling in your joints, heavier than normal or irregular menstrual periods, thinning hair, slowed heart rate, depression, impaired memory.

When hypothyroidism isn't treated, signs and symptoms can gradually become more severe. Constant stimulation of your thyroid gland to release more hormones may lead to an enlarged thyroid (goiter). In addition, you may become more forgetful, your thought processes may slow, or you may feel depressed.

Advanced hypothyroidism, known as myxedema, is rare, but when it occurs it can be life-threatening. Signs and symptoms include low blood pressure, decreased breathing, decreased body temperature, unresponsiveness and even coma. In extreme cases, myxedema can be fatal.

Although hypothyroidism most often affects middle-aged and older women, anyone can develop the condition, including infants. Initially, babies born without a thyroid gland or with a gland that does not work properly may have few signs and symptoms. When newborns do have problems with hypothyroidism, the problems may include: yellowing of the skin and whites of the eyes (jaundice). In most cases, this occurs when a baby's liver can't metabolize a substance called bilirubin, which normally forms when the body recycles old or damaged red blood cells: Frequent choking, a large, protruding tongue or a puffy appearance to the face. As the disease progresses, infants are likely to have trouble feeding and may fail to grow and develop normally. They may also have: constipation, poor muscle tone and excessive sleepiness.

When hypothyroidism in infants isn't treated, even mild cases can lead to severe physical and mental retardation.

In general, children and teens that develop hypothyroidism have the same signs and symptoms as adults do, but they may experience: poor growth, resulting in short stature, delayed development of permanent teeth, delayed puberty and poor mental development.

See your doctor if you are feeling tired for no reason or have any of the other signs or symptoms of hypothyroidism, such as dry skin, a pale, puffy face, constipation or a hoarse voice.

You will also need to see your doctor for periodic testing of your thyroid function if you have had previous thyroid surgery; treatment with radioactive iodine or anti thyroid medications; or radiation therapy to your head, neck or upper chest. However, it may take years or even decades before any of these therapies or procedures result in hypothyroidism.

If you have high blood cholesterol, talk to your doctor about whether hypothyroidism may be the cause. And if you are receiving in hormone therapy for hypothyroidism, schedule follow – up visits as often as your doctor recommends. Initially, it's important to make sure you're receiving the correct dose of medicine. And over time, the dose you need may change.

When your thyroid does not produce enough hormones, the balance of chemical reactions in your body can be upset. There can be a number of causes, including autoimmune disease, treatment for hypothyroidism, radiation therapy, thyroid surgery and certain medications.

Your thyroid is a small, butterfly-shaped gland situated at the base of the front of your neck, just below your Adam's apple. Hormones produced by the thyroid gland- triiodothyronine (T3) and thyroxine (T4) - have an enormous impact on your health, affecting all aspects of your metabolism. They maintain the rate at which your body uses fats and carbohydrates, help control your body temperature, influence your heart rate, and help regulate the production of proteins.

Hypothyroidism results when the thyroid gland fails to produce enough hormones. Hypothyroidism may be due to a number of factors, including:

Autoimmune disease- people who develop a particular inflammatory disorder known as Hashimoto's thyroiditis have the most common cause of hypothyroidism. Autoimmune disorders occur when your immune system produces antibodies that attack your own tissues. Sometimes this process involves your thyroid gland. Scientists are not sure why the body produces antibodies against itself. Some think a virus or bacterium might trigger the response, while others believe a genetic flaw may be involved. Most likely, autoimmune diseases result from more than one factor. But however it happens, these antibodies affect the thyroids ability to produce hormones.

People who produce too much thyroid hormone (hyperthyroidism) are often treated with radioactive iodine or anti-thyroid medications to reduce and normalize their thyroid function. However, in some cases, treatment of hyperthyroidism can result in permanent hypothyroidism.

Thyroid surgery, removing all or a large portion of your thyroid gland can diminish or halt hormone production. In that case, you will need to take thyroid hormone for the rest of your life.

Radiation therapy- used to treat cancers of the head and neck can affect your thyroid gland and may lead to hypothyroidism.

A number of medications can contribute to hypothyroidism. One such medication is lithium, which is used to treat certain psychiatric disorders. If you are taking medication, ask your doctor about its effect on your thyroid gland.

Congenital disease: some babies are born with a defective thyroid gland or no thyroid gland. In most cases, the thyroid gland didn't develop normally for unknown reasons, but some children have an inherited form of the disorder. Often infants with congenital hypothyroidism appear normal at birth. That's one reason why most states now require newborn thyroid screening.

Pituitary disorder: a relatively rare cause of hypothyroidism is the failure of the pituitary gland to produce enough thyroid stimulating hormone (TSH) – usually because of a benign tumor of the pituitary gland.

Pregnancy: Some women develop hypothyroidism during or after pregnancy (postpartum hypothyroidism), often because they produce antibodies to their own thyroid gland. Left untreated, hypothyroidism increases the risk of miscarriage, premature delivery and preeclampsia – a condition that causes a significant rise in a woman's blood pressure during the last three months of pregnancy. It can also seriously affect the developing fetus.

Iodine deficiency: The trace mineral iodine found primarily in seafood, seaweed, plants grown in iodine rich soil and iodized salt is essential for the production of thyroid hormones. In some parts of the world, iodine deficiency is common, but the addition of iodine to table salt has virtually eliminated this problem conversely, taking in too much iodine can cause hypothyroidism.

Although anyone can develop hypothyroidism, you're at an increased risk if you are a woman older than age 60, have an autoimmune disease, if you have a family history of thyroid disease, if you have other autoimmune diseases, such as rheumatoid arthritis or lupus, a chronic inflammatory condition, if you have been treated with radioactive iodine or anti-thyroid medications, received radiation to your neck or upper chest, have had thyroid surgery (partial thyroidectomy), have been pregnant or delivered a baby within the past six months.

Untreated hypothyroidism can lead to a number of health problems:

Goiter: constant stimulation of your thyroid to release more hormones may cause the gland to become larger – a condition known as a goiter, Hashimoto's thyroiditis is one of the most common causes of a goiter. Although generally not uncomfortable, a large goiter can affect your appearance and may interfere with swallowing or breathing.

Heart problems: Hypothyroidism may also be associated with an increased risk of heart disease, primarily because high levels of low density lipoprotein (LDL) – the bad cholesterol – can occur in people with an underactive thyroid. Even subclinical hypothyroidism, a mild or early form of hypothyroidism in which symptoms have not yet developed, can cause an increase in total cholesterol levels and impair the pumping ability of you heart. Hypothyroidism can also lead to an enlarged heart and heart failure.

Mental health issues: Depression may occur early in hypothyroidism and may become more severe over time. Hypothyroidism can also cause slowed mental functioning.

Peripheral neuropathy: Long – term uncontrolled hypothyroidism can cause damage to your peripheral nerves- the nerves that carry information from your brain and spinal cord to the rest of your body, for example, your arms and legs.

Signs and symptoms of peripheral neuropathy may include pain, numbness and tingling in the area affected by the nerve damage. It may also cause muscle weakness of loss of muscle control.

Myxedema: This rare, life threatening condition is the result of long-term undiagnosed hypothyroidism. Its signs and symptoms include intense cold intolerance and drowsiness followed by profound lethargy and unconsciousness. A myxedema coma may be triggered by sedatives, infection or other stress on your body. If you have signs or symptoms of myxedema, you need immediate emergency medical treatment.

Infertility: Low levels of thyroid hormone can interfere with ovulation, which impairs fertility. In addition, some of the causes of hypothyroidism – such as autoimmune disorder- can also impair fertility.

Birth defects: babies born to women with untreated thyroid disease may have a higher risk of birth defects than babies born to healthy mothers. These children are also more prone to serious intellectual and developmental problems. Infants with untreated hypothyroidism present at birth are at risk of serious problems with both physical and mental development. But if this condition is diagnosed within the first few months of life, the chances of normal development are excellent.

Because hypothyroidism is more prevalent in older women, some doctors recommend that older women be screened for the disorder during routine annual physical examinations. Some doctors also recommend that pregnant women or women thinking about becoming pregnant be tested for hypothyroidism. In general, your doctor may test for an underactive thyroid if you are feeling increasingly tired, have dry skin, constipation and weight gain, or have had previous thyroid problems or a goiter.

Diagnosis of hypothyroidism is based on your symptoms and the results of blood tests that measure the level of TSH and sometimes the level of the thyroid hormone thyroxine. A low level of thyroxine and high level of TSH indicate an underactive thyroid. That's because your pituitary produces more TSH in an effort to stimulate your thyroid gland into producing more thyroid hormone. In the past, doctors were not able to detect hypothyroidism until symptoms were fairly advanced. But by using the sensitive TSH test, doctors are able to diagnose thyroid disorders much earlier, often before you experience symptoms. Because the TSH test is the best screening test, your doctor will likely check TSH first ad follow with a thyroid hormone test if needed.

TSH test also play an important role in managing hypothyroidism. They help your doctor determine the right dosage of medication, both initially and over time. In addition, TSH tests are used to help diagnose a condition called subclinical hypothyroidism, which usually causes no outward signs or symptoms. In this condition, your have normal blood levels of triiodothyronine and thyroxine, but higher than normal levels of TSH.

Standard treatment for hypothyroidism involves daily use of the synthetic thyroid hormone levothyroxine (Levothroid, Synthroid, and others). This oral medication restores adequate hormone levels, reversing the signs and symptoms of hypothyroidism. One or two weeks after starting treatment, you will notice that you are feeling less fatigued. The medication also gradually lowers cholesterol levels elevated by the disease and may reverse any weight gain. Treatment with levothyroxine is usually life long, but because the dosage you need may change, your doctor is likely to check your TSH level every year.

To determine the right dosage of levothyroxine initially, your doctor generally checks your level of TSH after two to three months. Excessive amounts of the hormone can cause side effects. Such as: increased appetite, insomnia and heart palpitations. If you have coronary artery disease or severe hypothyroidism, your doctor may start treatment with a smaller amount of medication and gradually increase the dosage. Progressive hormone replacement allows your heart to adjust to the increase in metabolism. Levothyroxine causes virtually no side effects when used in the appropriate dose and is relatively inexpensive. If you change brands, let your doctor know to ensure you are still receiving the right dosage. Also don't skip doses or stop taking the drug because you are feeling better. If you do the symptoms of hypothyroidism will gradually return.

Certain medications, supplements and even some foods may affect your ability to absorb levothyroxine. Talk to your doctor if you eat large amounts of soy products or a high fiber diet or you take other medications, such as: iron supplements or multivitamins that contains iron, cholestyramine, and aluminum.

If you have subclinical hypothyroidism, discuss treatment with your doctor. For a relatively mild increase in TSH, you probably won't benefit from thyroid hormone therapy, and treatment could even be harmful. On the other hand, for a higher TSH level, thyroid hormones may improve your cholesterol level, the pumping ability of your heart and your energy level.

If you are worried about hypothyroidism I hope this helps and puts your mind at rest. I personally looked into this as my daughter has this and went through two surgeries to remove thyroid and goiter also had the radioactive iodine I thank God every day as she is a wonderful woman and mother of three beautiful girls.

Hyperthyroidism (overactive thyroid) is a condition in which your thyroid gland produces too much of the hormone thyroxine. It can accelerate your body's metabolism significantly, causing sudden weight loss, a rapid or irregular heartbeat, sweating and nervousness or irritability.

Several treatment options are available if you have hyperthyroidism. Doctors use anti-thyroid medications and radioactive iodine to slow the production of thyroid hormones. Sometimes, treatment of hyperthyroidism involves surgery to remove all or part of your thyroid gland. Although hyperthyroidism can be serious if you ignore it, most people respond well once it is diagnosed and treated.

Hyperthyroidism can mimic other health problems, which may make it difficult for your doctor to diagnose. It can also cause a wide variety of signs and symptoms, including: sudden weight loss, even when your appetite and the amount and type of food you eat remain the same or even increase, rapid heartbeat (tachycardia) commonly more than 100 beats a minute, irregular heartbeat (arrhythmia) or pounding of your heart (palpitations). Increased appetite, nervousness, anxiety and irritability, tremor usually a fine trembling in your hands and fingers, sweating, changes in menstrual patterns, increased sensitivity to heat, changes in bowel patterns, especially more frequent bowel movements, an enlarged thyroid gland (goiter), which may appear as a swelling at the base of your neck, fatigue, muscle weakness, difficulty sleeping, skin thinning, and fine brittle hair.

Older adults are more likely to have either no signs or symptoms or subtle ones, such as an increased heart rate, heat intolerance and a tendency to become tired during ordinary activities, medications called beta blockers, which are used to treat high blood pressure and other conditions, can mask many of the signs of hyperthyroidism.

A number of conditions, including Graves' disease, toxic adenoma, Plummer's disease, (toxic multinodular goiter) and thyroiditis, can cause hyperthyroidism.

Your thyroid is a butterfly – shaped gland at the base of the neck, just below your Adams apple. Although it weighs less than an ounce, the thyroid gland has an enormous impact on your health; every aspect of your metabolism is regulated by thyroid hormones.

Your thyroid gland produces two main hormones, thyroxine (T 4) and triodothyronine (T-3), that influence every cell in your body. They maintain the rate at which your body uses fats and carbohydrates, help control your body temperature, influence your heart rate, and help regulate the production of protein. Your thyroid also produces calcitonin, a hormone that helps regulate the amount of calcium in your blood.

The rate at which T-4 and T-3 are released is controlled by your pituitary gland and your hypothalamus- an area at the base of your brain that acts as a thermostat for your whole system. This is how it all works: the hypothalamus signals your pituitary gland to make a hormone called thyroid- stimulating hormone (TSH) the amount depends on how much T-4 and T-3 is in your blood. If you don't have enough T-4 and T-3 in your blood, your TSH will rise; if you have too much, your TSH level will fall. Finally your thyroid gland regulates its production of hormones.

Hyperthyroidism can lead to a number of complications:

Heart problems: some of the most serious complications of hyperthyroidism involve the heart. These include a rapid heart rate, a heart rhythm disorder called atrial fibrillation and congestive heart failure- a condition in which your heart can't circulate enough blood to meet your body's needs. These complications generally are reversible with appropriate treatment.

Brittle bones: untreated hyperthyroidism can also lead to weak, brittle bones (osteoporosis). The strength of your bones depends, in part, on the amount of calcium and other minerals they contain. Too much thyroid hormone interferes with you body's ability to incorporate calcium into your bones.

People with Graves' ophthalmopathy develop eye problems, including bulging, red or swollen eyes, sensitivity to light, and blurring or double vision. Untreated, severe eye problems can lead to vision loss.

Red swollen skin: In rare cases, people with Graves' disease develop Graves' dermopathy, which affects the skin, causing redness and swelling, often on the shins and feet.

Hyperthyroidism also places you at risk of Thyrotoxic crisis – a sudden intensification of your symptoms, leading to a fever, a rapid pulse and even delirium. If this occurs seek immediate medical care.

Hyperthyroidism, particularly Graves' disease, tends to run in families and is more common in women than in men. If another member of your family has a thyroid condition, talk with your doctor about what this may mean for your health and whether he or she has any recommendations for monitoring your thyroid functions.

I hope this gives you the information you may need on hyperthyroidism.

The next few chapters are very controversial: however, you just might learn something. And yes they have a lot to do with our children and your health.

Additives in food to avoid

Food additives have been used for centuries to enhance the appearance and flavor of food and prolong shelf life. However, do these food additives really add any value to your food? These additives find their way into our food to help ease processing, packaging, and storage, but how do we know what food additives are in that box of macaroni and cheese, and why does it have such a long shelf life? A typical household spends about 90 percent of their food budget on processed foods and in doing so, get exposed to a plethora of artificial food additives, many of which can have serious consequences to your health. Some are worse than others.

Artificial sweeteners= aspartame more popular known as NutraSweet and equal, is found in foods labeled "diet" or "sugar free". Aspartame is believed to be carcinogenic and accounts for more reports of adverse reactions than all other foods and food additives combined.

Aspartame is not your friend. Aspartame is a neurotoxin and carcinogen. Known to erode intelligence and affect short-term memory, the components of this toxic sweetener may lead to a wide variety of ailments including brain tumor, diseases like lymphoma, diabetes, multiple sclerosis, Parkinson's Alzheimer's fibromyalgia, and chronic fatigue, emotional disorders like depression and anxiety attacks, dizziness, headaches, nausea, mental confusion, migraines and seizures.

Acesulfame-k, a relatively new artificial sweetener found in baking goods, gum, and gelatin, has not been thoroughly tested and has been linked to kidney tumors, is the sweet taste worth it? I don't think so aspartame is found in diet or sugar-free sodas, diet coke, coke zero, jello and over gelatins, desserts, sugar free gum, drink mixes, baking goods, table top sweeteners, cereals, breath mints, pudding, Kool-Aid, ice tea, chewable vitamins, and toothpaste!

High fructose corn syrup is a highly – refined artificial sweetener which has become the number one source of calories. It is found in almost all processed foods. HFCS packs on pounds faster than any other ingredient, increases your LDL (bad cholesterol) levels, and contributes to the development of diabetes and tissue damage, among other harmful effects. It is found in most processed foods, bread, candy, flavored yogurts, salad dressings, canned vegetables and cereals.

Monosodium glutamate (MSG)= is an amino acid used as a flavor enhancer in soups, salad dressings, chips frozen entrees, and many restaurant foods. It is known as an excite-toxin which over excites cells to the point of damage or death. Studies show that regular consumption of MSG may result in adverse side effects which include depression, disorientation, eye damage, fatigue, headaches, and obesity, also affects the neurological pathways of the brain and disengage the" I'm full" function which explains the effects of weight gain.

It is found in Chinese food (Chinese restaurant syndrome) many snacks, chips, cookies, seasonings, most Campbell soup products, frozen dinners and lunch meats.

Trans- fats is used to enhance and extend the shelf life of food products, and is among the most dangerous substances that you can consume. Found in deep- fried foods and certain processed foods made with margarine or partially hydrogenated vegetable oils, trans fats are formed by a process called hydrogenation, numerous studies show that trans fats increase LDL cholesterol levels while decreasing HDL (good) cholesterol, increases the risk of heart attacks, heart disease, and strokes, and contributes to increased inflammation, diabetes, and other health problems. Oils and fat are now forbidden on the Danish market if they contain Trans- fatty acids exceeding 2 per cent, a move that effectively bans partially hydrogenated oils. Found in margarine, chips and crackers, baked goods, and fast foods.

Studies show that artificial colorings which are found in soda, fruit juices and salad dressings, may contribute to behavioral problems in children and lead to a significant reduction in IQ.

Animal studies have linked some food colorings to cancer. Found in candy, cereal, soft drinks, sport drinks and pet food.

Red dye banned in 1990 after 8 years of debate from use in many foods and cosmetics. This dye continues to be on the market until supplies run out. Has been proven to cause thyroid cancer and chromosomal damage in laboratory animals, may also interfere with brain – nerve transmission. Found in fruit cocktail, maraschino cherries, cherry pie- mix ice cream, candy, bakery products and more.

Sodium sulfite a preservative used in wine-making and other processed food

According to the FDA, approximately one in 100 people is sensitive to sulfites in food. The majority of these individuals are asthmatic, suggesting a link between asthma and sulfites. Individuals who are sulfite sensitive may experience headaches, breathing problems, and rashes. In severe cases, sulfites can actually cause death by closing down the airway altogether, leading to cardiac arrest.

Found in wine and dried fruit.

Sodium nitrate (or sodium nitrite) is used as a preservative, coloring, and flavoring in bacon, ham, hot dogs, lunch meats, corned beef, smoked fish, and other processed meats. This ingredient, which sounds harmless, is actually highly carcinogenic once it enters the human digestive system. There, it forms a variety of nitrosamine compounds that enter the bloodstream and wreak havoc with a number of internal organs: the liver and pancreas in particular. Sodium nitrite is widely regarded as a toxic ingredient. The USDA- actually tried to ban this additive in the 1970's but was vetoed by food manufacturers who complained they had no alternative for preserving packaged meat products.

Why does the industry still use it? Simple this chemical just happens to turn meats bright red. It's actually a color fixer, and makes old, dead meats appear fresh and vibrant. Found in hotdogs, bacon, ham, lunch meats, cured meats, corned beef, smoked fish and any other type of processed meat.

Butylated hydroxyanisole (BHA) and butylated hydroxytoluene (HBT) are preservatives found in cereals, chewing gum, potato chips and vegetable oils. This common preservative keeps foods from changing color, changing the flavor or becoming rancid. Affects the neurological system of the brain, alters behavior and has a potential to cause cancer. BHA and BHT are oxidants which form cancer-causing reactive compounds in your body. Also found in frozen sausages, enriched rice, lard, shortening candy and jello.

Sulfur additives are toxic and in the United States of America, the federal drugs administration has prohibited their use on raw fruit and vegetables. Adverse reactions include bronchial problems particularly in those prone to asthma,

Hypotension (low blood pressure): flushing tingling sensations or anaphylactic shock. It also destroys Vitamins B1 and E. not recommended for consumption by children. The international labour organization says to avoid sulfur dioxide if you suffer from conjunctivitis, bronchitis, emphysema, bronchial asthma or cardiovascular disease. Found in beer, soft drinks, dried fruit, juices, cordials, wine, vinegar, and potato products.

Potassium Bromate an additive used to increase volume in some white flour, bread, and rolls potassium bromate is known to cause cancer in animals. Even small amounts in bread can create problems for humans. Found in bread.

Other chemicals in your food

Anyone who has ever read a nutrition label knows that our food supply is full of hard –to – pronounce chemicals. Most are generally recognized as safe, as the food and drug administration like to say: however, a few have given scientists cause for concern.

Azodicarbonamide, for instance Subway announced that it would be removing the controversial chemical from its bread. Generally used for strengthening dough, Azodicarbonamide is also found in yoga mats and shoe soles, according to the centers for science in the public interest. One of the breakdown products is a recognized carcinogen. Although subway is going to remove Azodicarbonamide, there's a long list of other chemicals used in its bread calcium carbonate, calcium sulfate, ammonium sulfate, sodium stearoyl lactylate, potassium iodate and ascorbic acid,

Tartrazine and other food dyes; when Kraft announced that it would be removing No.5 (Tartrazine) and No 6 from certain varieties; of Macaroni & cheese products blue 1, green 3, red 40 and others have been loosely linked to everything from hyperactivity in children to cancer in lab animals.

Generally found in candy, beverages and baked goods. Color additives are also used in cosmetics. But you knew that! Did you also know about the ground up insects in your drinks?

Cochineal extract is an approved artificial dye derived from a small bug that lives on cactus plants in Mexico and South America. As long as you're not allergic, you're safe to drink up, according to the centers of science!

Chemicals we consume in our food and drink that should be banned

E numbers are bad we all know that and E290 is no exception. It sneaks its way into fizzy drinks bread and even your homemade cakes. This chemical is probably the worst of the lot, because if we don't stop producing it then we are headed for a global disaster. The scientific literature is quite clear on the subject; there are over a million peer-reviewed papers that describe the harmful effect it is having on our environment. And they put this stuff in our children's lemonade! 8-methyl-N-vannillyl -6-nonenamide with a name like that it's bound to be bad. It is used by the police to control rioters. But that doesn't stop it turning up in our favourite meals. In fact you have almost certainly suffered the consequences of an overzealous chef adding a bit too much of this stuff to your Saturday night post- pub curry or kebab. Do excessive sweating, burning sensations and indigestion sound familiar? Well that's good old 8-methyl-N-6-nonenamide for you. Would you believe they even put it in Chocolate?

Denatured protein: you may not know this but Alzheimer's disease, Parkinson's and CJD (the human version of mad cow disease) are all caused by proteins that have misfolded. Basically perfectly normal proteins get shape shifted into evil versions of themselves that then cause dreadful diseases.

DHMO fruit juice contains this chemical; that is also produced by rocket engines, think about that for a moment. The same stuff that comes shooting out of a rocket is in your fridge and you drink it for breakfast. Remember the Hindenburg disaster? The chemical reaction that destroyed the airship also produced DHMO. Fancy that in your refreshing glass of orange juice. It can even be found in mineral water, tap water, rainwater, in fact the oceans and lakes are literally full of the stuff.

NaC1 not one but two deadly poisons here: What do you think makes salty snacks so appealing? Nothing other than a delicious mix of a chemical warfare agent; used in the trenches of the First World War and an explosive metal. They put this chemical on our crisps, nuts and chips.

The overuse of antibiotics in food animals threatens public life

Antibiotics have been used since the 1940s and have led to a dramatic reduction in illness and death from infectious diseases. But according to the federal interagency task force on antimicrobial resistance "the intensive use of antimicrobial drugs has resulted in drug resistance that threatens to reverse the medical advances of the last seventy years". Since antibiotics have been used so widely and for so long; antibiotic resistance has become a major public health threat. In response, there has been a concerted effort by the centers of disease control and prevention and others to encourage doctors and patients to use antibiotics more wisely. Unfortunately, little progress has been made to reduce the use of antibiotics on farms, where most of these drugs are administered.

Approximately 80 percent of the antibiotics sold in the United States are used in meat and poultry production.

The vast majority is used on healthy animals to promote growth, or prevent disease in crowded or unsanitary conditions. The meat and poultry production industry argues, however, that there is no harm in this. They say that animal use contributes little if anything to the burden of human antibiotic resistance. A key question is; can antibiotic use in animals promote the development of hard to treat antibiotic superbugs that make people sick? And if so, are the illnesses rare and the risks theoretical, or could current usage in animals pose a serious threat to human health.

Consumers union has concluded that the threat to public health from the overuse of antibiotics in food animals is real and growing. Humans are at risk both due to potential presence of superbugs in meat and poultry, and to the general migration of superbugs into the environment, where they can transmit their genetic immunity to antibiotics, to other bacteria including bacteria that make people sick. Numerous health organizations, including world health organization agree and have called for a significant reduction in the use of antibiotics for animal food production. Scientific expert s for more than two decades have concluded that there is a connection between antibiotic use in animals and the loss of effectiveness of these drugs in human medicine. Thirty years ago the institute of medicine concluded that "the committee believes that important yet sparse data showed the flow of distinct salmonella clones from farm animals medicated with antibiotics In sub therapeutic concentrations, through food products, to humans who thus acquire salmonellosis.

Twenty years later the national research council concluded that a link can be demonstrated between the use of antibiotics in food animals, the development of resistant microorganisms in those animals and the zoonotic spread of pathogens to humans. Ten years later an expert workshop co-sponsored by the world health organization, concluded that there is clear evidence of adverse human health consequences due to resistant organisms resulting from non-human usage of antimicrobials. These consequences include infections that would not have otherwise occurred, increased frequency of treatment failures

(in some cases death) and increased severity of infections.in 2010 the U.S. food and drug administration, U.S. department of agriculture, and the CDC all testified before congress that there is a connection between the routine use of antibiotics for meat production and the declining effectiveness of antibiotics for people. Most recently in 2012 the FDA stated misuse and overuse of antimicrobial drugs creates selective evolutionary pressure that enables antimicrobial resistant bacteria to increase in numbers more rapidly than antimicrobial susceptible bacteria and thus increases the opportunity for individuals to become infected by resistant bacteria. Also in 2012 the FDA in its final rule banning certain extra label of cephalosporin antimicrobial drugs in certain food producing animals, stated in regard to antimicrobial drug use in animals, the agency considers the most significant risk to the public health associated with antimicrobial resistance to be human exposure to food containing antimicrobial- resistant bacteria resulting from the exposure of food producing animals to antimicrobials. Never the less, the livestock industry continues to argue that while antibiotic use may have something to do with antibiotic resistance in bacteria on the farm it is not an important human health issue, and little change in currant practices are needed.

Numerous studies have found that routine use of antibiotics on the farm promotes drug – resistant superbugs in those facilities. Some of the most dramatic evidence came as a result of FDA approval of flour quinolones – a class of antibiotics that includes Cipro (ciprofloxacin), which has been used in poultry production since 1995. By 1999 nearly 20 percent chicken breasts sampled contained ciprofloxacin – resistant Camplobacter, a disease –causing bacteria. After a long fight in the courts, FDA finally banned the use of the drug in 2005. At which point nearly 30 percent of coli found in chicken breasts were ciprofloxacin resistant, by 2010 resistance to ciprofloxacin had declined to 13.5 percent. The reason for this is when you feed antibiotics to animals; the bacteria in and around the animals are exposed to the drug, and many of them die. But there are always some that the drug can't kill, and those survive and proliferate. Voila, superbugs. While not disputing these facts, the industry argues essentially that what happens on the farm stays on the farm. There may be some superbugs there, but they don't affect people. There are two main routes, however, by which superbugs can leave the farm and infect humans. One is a direct route, in meat and poultry products, and the other is an indirect route the environment. Once they appear on the farm, superbugs most definitely move from the farm to the kitchen, via uncooked meat and poultry. Consumer reports tests of chicken, revealed widespread presence of antibiotic- resistant pathogens in retail poultry products; more than two thirds of chicken samples were contaminated with salmonella and/or campylobacter, and more than 60 percent of those bacteria were resistant to one or more antibiotics.

The industry argues that even this is not a concern because people know how to cook poultry thoroughly. Indeed they do, but packages can drip in the refrigerator, or cutting boards can become contaminated, as well as other problems.

There is no good data on how frequently this causes illness, especially difficult-to treat- illness, because most people just ride out an infection and it fades into the background of the estimated 48 million cases of food borne illness we have annually. Occasionally a superbug outbreak is serious to command the attention of the center for disease control. One such case occurred in 2011, in which ground turkey was linked to 136 illnesses and one death, all caused by a strain of salmonella resistant to four different antibiotics, ampicillin, streptomycin, tetracycline and gentamicin. 36 million pounds of ground turkey were recalled. Another case was ground beef in 2011 nineteen infections and seven hospitalizations, all caused by a strain of salmonella resistant to multiple antibiotics, including amoxicillin, ampicillin, ceftriaxone, cefoxitin, kanamycin, streptomycin and sulfisoxazole.

Superbugs can spread beyond the farm and threaten public health through environment transmission. This can happen in various ways, particularly via workers, or farm runoff. Once farm-raised superbugs make it off the farm, they can exchange genetic material and give their resistance to other bacteria, even of other species. This can happen in lakes, wild animals, and even in the human digestive tract. Workers are particularly likely to pick up resistant bacteria from animals and take them elsewhere. A study of poultry workers, found they were 32 times more likely to carry gentamicin-resistant Escherichia coli; and more than five times more likely to carry multi-drug resistant E. coli, a study performed in the Midwest found methicillin- resistant Staphylococcus aureus (MRSA) in 70 percent of the pigs and 64 percent in the workers and one facility, while no MRSA was found in pigs or workers in another state, strongly suggesting that MRSA strain moves between pigs and humans. Indeed a careful genetic analysis has found that a particular MRSA found in pigs originated as a methicillin- susceptible S. aureus (MSSA) in humans, jumped into pigs, where it acquired resistance to methicillin and tetracycline, and then jumped back into humans, where its known as livestock – associated MRSA (LA-MRSA) is quite prevalent in the Netherlands where it is responsible for over 20% of all MRSA20.

However, resistant bacteria can also escape from a large livestock operation

(often known as a confined animal feeding operation) by a number of routes, including via manure applied to fields as fertilizer, form truck transporting animals, the wind leaving hog facilities, or even via flies attracted to the manure which can pick up and transmit resistant bacteria. A recent released study found that antibiotic resistance genes were 10,000 times higher in river sediments downstream from larger feedlots (ones with 10,000 cattle) compared to river sediments upstream from such feedlots. The same study found these same antibiotic resistance genes were only 1,000 times higher from sewage treatment plants that discharge ten million gallons of effluent per day, compared to pristine sediments.

Bacteria in many environments can readily exchange genes coding for antibiotic resistance with neighboring bacteria. Antibiotic resistance genes are often located on mobile genetic elements, especially plasmids, transposons, which can easily move between bacteria of the same or different species, which facilitates the spread of resistance to multiple drugs by multiple types of bacteria.

Use of antibiotics on the farm most definitely poses a risk to human health.

Antibiotic use can promote creation of superbugs which can contaminate meat and poultry and cause hard-to – cure diseases in people.

Superbugs can also exit the farm; (farm workers, wind, runoff, and wildlife). Even if they don't immediately cause illness, bacteria are uniquely equipped to exchange genetic immunity via their plasmids, with other bacteria wherever they encounter them.

ANTIBIOTICS AND THE MEAT WE EAT

Scientist at the food and drug administration systematically monitor the meat and poultry sold in supermarkets around the country for the presence of disease causing bacteria that are resistant to antibiotics. These food products are bellwethers that tell us how bad the crisis of antibiotic resistance is getting, and they're telling us it's getting worse. This is only part of the story. While the F.D.A. can see what kinds of antibiotic-resistant bacteria are coming out of livestock facilities, the agency does not know enough about the antibiotics that are being fed to these animals. This is a major public health problem, because giving healthy livestock these drugs breeds superbugs that can infect people. We need to know more about the use of antibiotics in the production of our meat and poultry. The results could be a matter of life and death. In 2011, drug makers sold nearly 30 million pounds of antibiotics for livestock- the largest amount yet recorded and about 80 percent of all reported antibiotic sales that year. The rest was for human health care. I don't know much more except that, rather than healing sick animals, these drugs are often fed to animals at low levels to make them grow faster and to suppress diseases that arise because they live in dangerously close quarters on top of one another's waste.

It may sound counterintuitive, but feeding antibiotics to livestock at low levels may do the most harm. When Alexander Fleming got the Nobel Prize in 1945 for his discovery of penicillin, he warned that "there is the danger that the ignorant man may easily under dose himself and by exposing his microbes to nonlethal quantities of the drug make them resistant." He probably could not have imagined that, one day, we would be doing this to billions of animals in factory like facilities. The F.D.A. started testing retail meat and poultry for antibiotic- resistant bacteria in 1996. The agency's most recent report on superbugs in our meat, released in 2011 covering retail purchases, was 82 pages long and broke down its results by four different kinds of meat and poultry products and dozens of species and strains of bacteria. It was not until 2008 that congress required companies to tell the F.D.A. the quantity of antibiotics they sold for use in agriculture. The agency's report on sales for 2011 was four pages long including the cover and two pages of boilerplate. There was no information on how these drugs were administered or to which animals and why.

There is more than enough scientific evidence to justify curbing the rampant use of antibiotics for livestock, yet the food and drug industries are not only fighting proposed legislation to reduce these practices, they also oppose collecting the data. Unfortunately, the Senate Committee on health, education, labor and pensions, as well as the F.D.A., is aiding and abetting them.

The senate committee recently approved the animal drug user fee act, a bill that would authorize the F.D.A. to collect fees from veterinary – drug makers to finance the agency's review of their products. Public health experts had urged the committee to require drug companies to provide more detailed antibiotic sales data to the agency. Yet the F.D.A. stood by silently as the committee declined to act, rejecting a modest proposal; that required the agency to report data it already collects but does not disclose. In the house, Representatives have introduced a more comprehensive measure. It would not only authorize the F.D.A. to collect more detailed data from drug companies, but would also require food producers to disclose how often they fed antibiotics to animals at low levels to make them grow faster and to offset poor conditions. This information would be particularly valuable to the F.D.A., which asked drug makers to voluntarily stop selling antibiotics for these purposes. The agency has said it would mandate such action if those practices persisted, but it has no data to determine whether the voluntary policy is working. Combating resistance requires monitoring both the prevalence of antibiotic- resistant bacteria in our food, as well as the use of antibiotics on livestock.

In human medicine, hospitals increasingly track resistance rates and antibiotic prescription rates to understand how the use of these drugs affects resistance. We need to cover both sides of this equation in agriculture, too. I realize that not everyone is as convinced as I am that feeding low-dose antibiotics to animals is a recipe for disaster. But most, if not all of you, recognize that we are facing an antibiotic resistance crisis.

It is now 2016 and for the first time, researchers have found a person in the United States carrying bacteria resistant to antibiotic of last resort, an alarming development that the top U.S. public health official says could signal "the end of the road" for antibiotics. The antibiotic –resistant strain was found last month in the urine of a 49 year old woman. Defence department researchers determined that she carried a strain of E. coli resistant to the antibiotic colistin, according to a study published in Antimicrobial Agents and Chemotherapy, a publication of the American Society for Microbiology. The authors wrote that the discovery "heralds the emergence; of a truly pan-drug resistant bacteria."

Colistin is the antibiotic of last resort for particularly dangerous types of superbugs, including a family of bacteria known as carbapenem –resistant Enterobacteriaceae, or CRE, which health officials have dubbed "nightmare bacteria." In some instances, these superbugs kill up to 50 percent of patients who become infected. The Centers for Disease Control and Prevention has called CRE among the country's most urgent public health threats. Health officials said the one case, by itself, is not cause for panic. The strain found in the woman is treatable with some other antibiotics. But researchers worry that the antibiotic-resistant gene found in the bacteria, known as mcr-1 could spread to other types of bacteria that can already evade other types of antibiotics.

It is the first time this colistin- resistant strain has been found in a person in the United States. In November 2015 health officials worldwide reacted with alarm when Chinese and British researchers reported finding the colistin-resistant strain in pigs, raw pork meat and in a small number of people in China. The deadly strain was later discovered in Europe, Africa, South America and Canada.

It basically shows us that the end of the road isn't very far away for antibiotics- that "we may be in a situation where patients in our intensive-care units, or patients getting urinary tract infections for which we do not have antibiotics," CDC Director, said in an interview, this is not where we need to be.

Researchers at the U.S. Department of Agriculture and the Health and Humans Services Department reported that testing of hundreds of livestock and retail meats turned up the same colistin-resistant bacteria in a sample from a pig intestine in the United States. The USDA said it is working to determine the pig's farm of origin. Colistin is widely used in Chinese livestock, and this use probably led bacteria to evolve and gain a resistance to the drug. That probably leaped from livestock to human microbes through food.

Food handlers may be at higher risk. In places like China, where live animal markets are often in close proximity to food stalls, it may be more likely for the bacteria to spread from animals to humans. We don't need to panic, but the research does tell us that this concerning gene is in the United States. Infectious disease experts call for speedier action to curb the overuse of antibiotics in livestock. Scientists rang the alarm bell in November, but not enough attention was paid. Now we find that this gene has made its way into pigs and people in the U.S. if our leaders were waiting to act until they could see the cliff's edge. I hope this opens their eyes to what lies before us.

Scientists and public health officials have long warned that if the resistant bacteria continue to spread, treatment options could be seriously limited. Routine operations could become deadly. Minor infections could become life- threatening crises. Pneumonia could be more difficult to treat. Doctors have been forced to rely on colistin as a last – line of defense against antibiotic- resistant bacteria. The drug is hardly ideal. It is more than a half a century old and can seriously damage a patient's kidneys; and yet because doctors have run out of weapons to fight a growing number of infections that evade more modern antibiotics. It has become a critical tool in fighting off some of the most tenacious infections.

Back in the 1980s most people who acquired a bacterial infection would receive antibiotics and just like magic the infection would be gone. To-day is a very different picture now we are dealing on a daily basis with stubborn, hard to treat and sometimes fatal infections that have become immune to, or have even resulted from the very antibiotics that used to work so beautifully. At least four or five people are in the ICU units fighting off superbugs these patients are kept in isolation, the nurses and doctors who treat them use disposable gowns, gloves, masks and eyewear protection each time they enter the room, and wash their hands dozens of times a day. The patients, who must undergo complex treatment and endure long hospital stays, have a higher risk of long –term disability, and some die.

Figuring out the new reality is a huge issue. Hospitals do not want to publicize their problem with antimicrobial-resistant infections.

A 2013 survey of 176 acute hospitals found that one in 12 adult patients is either infected or colonized with the three most common superbugs.

If they're infected, they are already sick with it; if they are colonized, they may become sick or pass it to others. The problem of antimicrobial resistance goes far beyond hospitals. It is an important, pervasive and global issue says a director of infection control there isn't anywhere you can look where resistance isn't an issue. "In hospitals, out in the community, foodborne illnesses, sexually transmitted infections, tuberculosis, malaria-resistance is everywhere." Conservative estimates suggest that more than two million people in North America get sick every year with infections resistant to antimicrobial drugs, which include mostly antibiotics but also antiparasitics, antivirals and antifungals.

About 25,000 die from these infections, and many more die from conditions complicated by such an infection. More than a quarter of North American cases of salmonella, caused from eating contaminated food are resistant to one or more antibiotics. About one in five urinary tract infections is now resistant to the sulfa drugs that were once a reliable cure. While gonorrhoea was once easily treated; now as many as 60 per cent of cases worldwide may be caused by multi-drug resistant strains. Globally there are 630,000 cases of multi-drug resistant tuberculosis in 84 countries.

Antimicrobial – resistant infections can still be treated, but when first- line drugs the most narrowly targeted ones with the fewest side effects don't work doctors must turn to more broad –spectrum second-line drugs, which may be less effective, cost more and have worse side effects.

If those fail, doctors try even harsher third –line drugs. The cost, both human and financial, are enormous, the U.S. Centers for Disease Control and Prevention estimates that antibiotic resistance costs that country's economy up to $55 billion a year due to increased health-care costs and lost productivity. It's one of the most important public health concerns of the 21st century, especially with health-care systems already heavily burdened with non- communicable illnesses such as heart disease, diabetes and cancer. The world health organization (WHO) in August 2013 warned, if we begin to add on top of that a lot of untreatable or

Difficult-to treat infections, we really are going to bring some of these health systems to the brink.

In Canada, an estimated 250,000 patients each year develop difficult infections, costing our health-care system an extra $1 billion annually, and despite their treatment several thousand of these patients will die. "With these superbugs, we have now reached an age where some patients' infections are resistant to all antibiotics, for those patients there are no usable antibiotics left."

During much of the 20th century, antibiotics were considered wonder drugs that would rid the world of all infections. What happened? Why have many of them stopped working? There are several reasons, starting with the bacteria themselves. These creatures, which have been around for billions of years longer than humans, are perfect examples of evolution in action. They evolve quickly to survive any threat, including a drug designed to kill them. There are so many bacteria – billions- that new mutations arise often. For instance, if some bacteria develop membranes that drugs can't get through, those will survive drug treatment and proliferate. Others may produce potent enzymes that inactivate the antibiotic. Still others may acquire resistance genes from different bacteria or even different species such as viruses. It is not that you become resistant to an antibiotic; it is that the bacteria do. It's nature's inevitable defence strategy: survival of the fittest.

Humans have unwittingly sped up this natural selection process through overuse of antibiotics. (The more we take antibiotics, the more quickly bacteria evolve.) Antibiotics are among the most commonly prescribed drugs worldwide. The latest figures from 2013 report on the state of public health in Canada shows that for every 1,000 Canadians, there are 670 prescriptions for oral antimicrobials filled every year. The U.S. Centers for Disease Control and Prevention estimates that up to 50 per cent of all antibiotics prescribed are unnecessary (in many cases. We would be better without them) or they are not optimally effective as prescribed; and that's just in people.

More than three – quarters of antimicrobials in Canada are given to food animals such as cattle, pigs, chickens and fish. Ninety per cent of the time the drugs are given to healthy animals to help prevent infections or promote growth. (For reasons not well understood, antibiotics help animals grow faster on less food and make them market- ready sooner.) Sometimes antibiotics for animals are the same ones used in people, and resistant bacteria can travel from animals to humans.

It was only a matter of time for us to build up a resistance to antibiotics especially when we are digesting it in our food, I guess that time is now.

The WHO says when healthy chickens receive tetracycline, within 36 hours their excrement contains resistant E.coli, a common cause of infection in people, a 2013 Mount Sinai study in Ontario and Alberta found that the risk of resistant E.coli was highest near properties housing livestock. Resistant bacteria are even turning up in bottled mineral water.

The European Union banned the use of antibiotics as growth promoters in animals in 2006, and the U.S. Food and Drug Administration began implementing a voluntary plan with the American agricultural industry in late 2013. But in Canada, not only do we lack any official guidelines or policies to manage antimicrobial use in animals, but we are one of the few industrialized countries where farmers can buy over-the counter antibiotics simply to promote growth in animals, without a veterinarian's prescription. In 2013 the Ontario Medical Association called on federal and provincial governments to crack down on antibiotic overuse in farming, with no results yet.

While overuse of antimicrobials is a danger, so is under-doing dosing. Scientists have known for decades that using too little of an antibiotic can hasten resistance. If you take too low a dose of an antibiotic or stop it too soon, you may kill of many of the bacteria that are causing the infection but leave stragglers that may be slightly resistant. These can survive, multiply, increase their resistance with each new generation, eventually outnumber the non-resistant bacteria, and be passed to another person. So the same antibiotic may not work the next time you or a family member needs it.

You need more information about this, but doctors need to be reminded as well family physicians and community doctors all across Canada need to be educated about the importance of this issue.

Resistance is a serious situation, but certainly not a hopeless one. It is a bit like global warming. It's not an immediate catastrophe, but it could become one if we don't do something soon. There is no single solution to the problem of antimicrobial resistance. Researchers around the world are pursuing a variety of strategies. One of them involves antimicrobial stewardship programs. Now mandatory in all North America's acute care hospitals, these programs aim to optimize antibiotic use to maximize their effects and minimize their harm. They generally involve surveillance screening of all patients for infection, regardless of why they come to hospital, and monitoring all antibiotic use. Only infectious disease specialists can approve certain broad –spectrum antibiotics. Another way researchers are tackling transmission of infection is by prioritizing prevention. Probably the main route of transfer of infection is on the hands of health-care workers.

Improving cleaning methods and increasing hand washing are essential, but they can cause their own problems. Washing and using hand sanitizers will dry the hands and cause cracks and bleeding, leaving them open for infection. Sinks in hospital rooms can actually increase infections because bacteria like moisture.

Because of all the things a doctor, nurse, or technician has to touch – doors, beds, switches, equipment, pens, wheelchairs, computer keyboards, and patients; it is impossible to keep hands constantly clean. Industrial antibacterial cleansers and detergents, for cleaning rooms, don't significantly reduce infections and may even contribute to antimicrobial resistance. With resistance such a global challenge, why don't we just create new antibiotics? Bringing a new drug to market can take more than 10 years and cost a billion dollars.

Pharmaceutical companies, who must answer to shareholders, are more inclined to invest in developing a drug that people take daily- such as for high blood pressure, high cholesterol or arthritis- than an antibiotic that people take as rarely as possible. FOOD SAFETY these questions and answers where prepared by WHO (world health organization); With regard to the nature and safety of genetically modified food.

What are genetically modified foods?

Genetically modified organisms (GMOs) can be defined as organisms in which the genetic material (DNA) has been altered in a way that does not occur naturally. The technology is often called modern biotechnology or gene technology, sometimes also recombinant DNA technology or genetic engineering. It allows selected individual genes to be transferred from one organism into another, also between non- related species. Such methods are used to create GM plants which are then used to grow GM food crops.

Why are GM foods produced?

GM foods are developed and marketed because there is some perceived advantage either to the producer or consumer of these foods. This is meant to translate into a product with a lower price, greater benefit in terms of durability or nutritional value or both. Initially GM seed developers wanted their products to be accepted by producers so have concentrated on innovations that farmers (and the food industry more generally) would appreciate. The initial objective for developing plants based on GM organisms was to improve crop protection. The GM crops currently on the market are mainly aimed at an increased level of crop protection through the introduction of resistance against plant diseases caused by insects or viruses or through increased tolerance towards herbicides.

Insect resistance is achieved by incorporating into the food plant the gene for toxin production from the bacterium Bacillus thuringiensis (BT). This toxin is currently used as a conventional insecticide in agriculture and is safe for human consumption. GM crops that permanently produce this toxin have been shown to require lower quantities of insecticides in specific situations, where pest pressure is high. Virus resistance is achieved through the introduction of a gene from certain viruses which cause disease in plants. Virus resistance makes plants less susceptible to diseases caused by such viruses, resulting in higher crop yields. Herbicide tolerance is achieved through the introduction of a gene from a bacterium conveying resistance to some herbicides. In situations where weed pressure is high, the use of such crops has resulted in a reduction in the quantity of the herbicides used.

Are GM foods assessed differently from traditional foods?

Generally consumers consider that traditional foods that have been eaten for thousands of years are safe. When new foods are developed by natural methods, some of the existing characteristics of foods can be altered, either in a positive or a negative way national food authorities may be called upon to examine traditional foods, but this is not always the case. Indeed new plants developed through traditional breeding techniques may not be evaluated rigorously using risk assessment techniques. With GM foods most national authorities consider that specific assessments are necessary. Specific systems have been set up for the rigorous evaluation of GM organisms and GM foods relative to both human health and the environment. Similar evaluations are generally not performed for traditional foods. There is a significant difference in the evaluation process prior to marketing for these two groups of food. One of the objectives of the WHO food safety programme is to assist national authorities in the identification of foods that should be subject to risk assessment, including GM foods, and to recommend the correct assessments.

How are the potential risks to human health determined?

The safety assessment of GM foods generally investigates: direct health effects (toxicity), tendencies to provoke allergic reaction (allergenicity), specific components thought to have nutritional or toxic properties, the stability of the inserted gene, nutritional effects associated with genetic modification and any unintended effects which could result from the gene insertion.

What are the main concerns for human health?

While theoretical discussions have covered a broad range of aspects, the three main issues are tendencies to provoke allergic reaction, gene transfer an outcrossing. Allergic reaction, as a matter of principle the transfer of genes from commonly allergenic foods is discouraged unless it can be demonstrated that the protein product of the transferred gene is not allergenic. While traditionally developed foods are not generally tested for allergic reactions, protocols for tests for GM foods have been evaluated by the food and agriculture organization of the United Nations and WHO. No allergic effects have been found relative to GM foods currently on the market. Gene transfer from GM foods to cells of the body or to bacteria in the gastrointestinal tract would cause concern if the transferred genetic material adversely affects human health. This would be particularly relevant if antibiotic resistance genes, used in creating GMOs, were to be transferred. Although the probability of transfer is low, the use of technology without antibiotic resistance genes has been encouraged by a recent FAO/WHO expert panel. Outcrossing: The movement of genes from GM plants into conventional crops or related species in the wild (referred to as outcrossing) as well as the mixing of crops derived from conventional seeds with those grown using GM crops, may have an indirect effect on food safety and food security. The risk is real, as was shown when traces of a maize type which was only approved for feed use appeared in maize products for human consumption in the United States of America. Several countries have adopted strategies to reduce mixing, including a clear separation of the fields within which GM crops and conventional crops are grown. Feasibility and methods for post-marketing monitoring of GM food products, for the continued surveillance of the safety of GM food products, are under discussion.

How is a risk assessment for the environment performed?

Environmental risk assessments cover both the GMO concerned and the potential receiving environment. The assessment process includes evaluation of the characteristics of the GMO and its effect and stability in the environment, combined with ecological characteristics of the environment in which the introduction will take place. The assessment also includes unintended effects which could result from the insertion of the new gene.

What are the concerns for the environment?

Issues of concern include: the capability of the GMO to escape and potentially introduce the engineered genes into wild populations; the persistence of the gene after the GMO has been harvested; the susceptibility of non-target organisms (e.g. insects which are not pests) to the gene product; the stability of the gene; the reduction in the spectrum of other plants including loss of biodiversity; and increased use of chemicals in agriculture. The environmental safety aspects of GM crops vary considerably according to local conditions. Current investigations focus on: the potentially detrimental effect on beneficial insects or a faster induction of resistant insects; the potential generation of new plant pathogens; the potential detrimental consequences for plant biodiversity and wild life, and a decreased use of the important practice of crop rotation in certain local situations; and the movement of herbicide resistance genes to other plants.

Are GM foods safe?

Different GM organisms include different genes inserted in different ways. This means that individual GM foods and their safety should be assessed on a case –by – case basis and that it is not possible to make general statements on the safety of all GM foods. GM foods currently available on the international market have passed risk assessments and are not likely to present risks for human health. In addition no effects on human health have been shown as a result of the consumption of such foods by the general population in the countries where they have been approved. Continuous use of risk assessments based on the Codex principles and where appropriate, including post market monitoring, should form the basis for evaluating the safety of GM foods.

How are GM foods regulated nationally?

The way governments have regulated GM foods varies. In some countries GM foods are not yet regulated. Countries which have legislation in place focus primarily on assessment of risk for consumer health. Countries which have provisions for GM foods usually also regulate GMOs in general, taking into account health and environmental risks, as well as control- and trade- related issues (such as potential testing and labelling regimes). In view of the dynamics of the debate on GM foods, legislation is likely to continue to evolve.

What kind of GM foods are on the market internationally?

All GM crops available on the international market today have been designed using one of three basic traits: resistance to insect damage; resistance to viral infections and tolerance towards certain herbicides. All the genes used to modify crops are derived from microorganisms.

What happens when GM foods are traded internationally?

No specific international regulatory systems are currently in place. However, several international organizations are involved in developing protocols for GMOs. The codex Aliment Arius commission is the joint FAO/WHO body responsible for compiling the standards, codes of practice; guidelines and recommendations that constitute the codes aliment Arius the international food code. Codex is developing principles for the human health risk analysis of GM foods. The premise of these principles dictates a premarket assessment, performed on a case-by case-basis and including an evaluation of both direct effects (from the inserted gene) and unintended effects (that may arise as a consequence of insertion of the new gene). The principles are at an advanced stage of development and are expected to be adopted in 2003. Codex principles do not have a binding effect on national legislation, but are referred to specifically in the sanitary and phytosanitary agreement of the world trade organization and can be used as a reference in case of trade disputes. The Cartagena protocol biosafety environmental treaty legally binding for its parties regulates trans-boundary movements of living modified organisms. GM foods are within the scope of the protocol only if they contain GMOs that are capable of transferring or replicating genetic material. The cornerstone of the CPB is a requirement that exporters seek consent from importers before the first shipment of GMOs intended for release into the environment. The protocol will enter into force in 90 days after the 50th country has ratified it, which may be in early 2003 in view of the accelerated depositions registered since June 2002.

Have GM products on the international market passed a risk assessment?

GM products that are currently on the international market have all passed risk assessments in general follow the same basic principles, including an assessment of environmental and human health risk. These assessment are thorough, they have not indicated any risk to human health.

Why has there been concern about GM foods among some politicians, public interest groups and consumers, especially in Europe?

Since the first introduction on the market in the mid-1990s of a major GM food (herbicide- resistant soybeans), there has been increasing concern about such food among politicians, activists and consumers, especially in Europe several factors are involved. In the late 1980s early 1990s the results of decades of molecular research reached the public domain. Until that time, consumers were generally not very aware of the potential of this research.

In the case of food, consumers started to wonder about safety because they perceive that modern biotechnology is leading to the creation of new species. Consumers frequently ask, what is in it for me.

Where medicines are concerned, many consumers more readily accept biotechnology as beneficial for their health (medicines with improved treatment potential). In the case of the first GM foods introduced onto the European market, the products were of no apparent direct benefit to consumers not cheaper, no increased shelf-life, and no better taste).

The potential for GM seeds to result in bigger yields per cultivated area should lead to lower prices; however, public attention has focused on the risk side of the risk – benefit equation.

Consumer confidence in the safety of food supplies in Europe has decreased significantly as a result of a number of food scares that took place in the second half of the 1990s that are unrelated to GM foods. This has also had an impact on discussions about the acceptability of GM foods. Consumers have questioned the validity of risk assessments, both with regard to consumer health and environmental risks, focusing in particular on long – term effects.

Other topics for debate by consumer organizations have included allergenicity and antimicrobial resistance. Consumer concerns have triggered a discussion on the desirability of labelling GM foods, allowing an informed choice. At the same time, it has proved difficult to detect traces of GMOs in foods: this means that very low concentrations often cannot be detected.

How has this concern affected the marketing of GM foods in the European Union?

The public concerns about GM food and GMOs in general have had a significant impact on the marketing of GM products in the European Union. In fact, they have resulted in the so-called moratorium on approval of GM products to be placed on the market. Marketing of GM food and GMOs in general are the subject of extensive legislation. Community legislation has been in place since the early 1990s. The procedure for approval of the release of GMOs into the environment is rather complex and basically requires agreement between the member States and the European Commission.

The new directive also foresees mandatory monitoring of long-term effects associated with the interaction between GMOs and the environment. Labelling in the EU is mandatory for products derived from modern biotechnology or products containing GM organisms. Legislation also addresses the problem of accidental contamination of conventional food by GM material. It introduces a 1% minimum threshold for DNA or protein resulting from genetic modification, below which labelling is not required. In 2001, the European commission adopted two new legislative proposals on GMOs. Concerning traceability, reinforcing current labelling rules; and streamlining the authorization procedure for GMOs: in food and feed and for their deliberate release into the environment.

The European commission is of the opinion that these new proposals, building on existing legislation, aim to address the concerns of member States and to build consumer confidence in the authorization of GM products. The commission expects that adoption of these proposals will pave the way for resuming the authorization of new GM products in the EU.

What is the state of public debate on GM foods in other regions of the world?

The release of GMOs into the environment and the marketing of GM foods have resulted in a public debate in many parts of the world. This debate is likely to continue, probably in the broader context of other uses of biotechnology (in human medicine) and their consequences for human societies. Even though the issues under debate are usually very similar (costs and benefits, safety issues) the outcome of the debate differs from country to country. On issues such as labelling and traceability of GM foods as a way to address consumer concerns, there is no consensus to date. This has become apparent during discussions within the commission over the past few years. Despite the lack of consensus on these topics, significant progress has been made on the harmonization of views concerning risk assessment; and the provisions of the Cartagena protocol on biosafety also reveal a growing understanding at the international level.

Most recently, the humanitarian crisis in southern Africa has drawn the attention to the use of GM food as food aid in emergency situations. A number of governments in the region raised concerns relating to environmental and food safety fears. Although workable solutions have been found for distribution of milled grain in some countries, others have restricted the use of GM food aid and obtained commodities which do not contain GMOs.

Are people's reactions related to the different attitudes to food in various regions of the world?

Depending on the region of the world, people often have different attitudes to food. In addition to nutritional value, food often has societal and historical connotations, and in some instances may have religious importance. Technological modification of food and food production can evoke a negative response among consumers, especially in the absence of good communication on risk assessment efforts and cost/benefit evaluations.

Are there implications for the rights of farmers to own their crops?

Intellectual property rights are likely to be an element in the debate on GM foods, with an impact on the rights of farmers. Intellectual property rights, especially patenting obligations of the trips agreement (an agreement under the world trade organization concerning trade-related aspects of intellectual property rights) have been discussed in the light of their consequences on the further availability of a diversity of crops. In the context of the related subject of the use of gene technology in medicine, WHO has reviewed the conflict between IPRs and equal access to genetic resources and the sharing of benefits? The review has considered potential problems of monopolization and doubts about new patent regulations in the field of genetic sequences in human medicine. Such considerations are likely to also affect the debate on GM foods.

Why are certain groups concerned about the growing influence of the chemical industry on agriculture?

Certain groups are concerned about what they consider to be an undesirable level of control of seed markets by a few chemical companies. Sustainable agriculture and biodiversity benefit most from the use of a rich variety of crops, both in terms of good crop protection practices as well as from the perspective of society at large and the values attached to food. These groups fear that as a result of the interest of the chemical industry in seed markets, the range of varieties used by farmers may be reduced mainly to GM crops. This would impact on the food basket of a society as well as in the long run on crop protection (for example, with the development of resistance against insect pests and tolerance of certain herbicides). The exclusive use of herbicide- tolerant GM crops would also make the farmer dependent on these chemicals. These groups fear a dominant position of the chemical industry in agricultural development, a trend which they do not consider to be sustainable.

And they were right: should have listened to the farmers.

What further developments can be expected in the area of GMOs?

Future GM organisms are likely to include plants with improved disease or drought resistance, crops with increased nutrient levels, fish species with enhanced growth characteristics and plants or animals producing pharmaceutically important proteins such as vaccines. At the international level, the response to new developments can be found in the expert consultations organized by FAO and WHO in 2000 and 2001, and the subsequent work of the Codex ad hoc task force on foods derived from Biotechnology. This work has resulted in an improved and harmonized framework for the risk assessment of GM foods in general. Specific questions, such as the evaluation of allergenicity of GM foods or the safety of foods derived from GM microorganisms, have been covered and an expect consultation organized by FAO and WHO will focus on foods derived from GM animals in 2003.

What is WHO doing to improve the evaluation of GM foods?

WHO will take an active role in relation to GM foods, primarily for two reasons?

1 On the grounds that public health could benefit enormously from the potential of biotechnology, for example, from an increase in the nutrient content of foods, decreased allergenicity and more efficient food production; and (2) based on the need to examine the potential negative effects on human health of the consumption of food produced through genetic modification, also at the global level. It is clear that modern technologies must be thoroughly evaluated if they are to constitute a true improvement in the way food is produced. Such evaluations must be holistic and all-inclusive, and cannot stop at the previously separated, non-coherent systems of evaluation focusing solely on human health or environmental effects in isolation. Work is therefore under way in; WHO to present a broader view of the evaluation of GM foods in order to enable

the consideration of other important factors. This more holistic evaluation of GM organisms and GM products will consider not only safety but also food security, social and ethical aspects, access and capacity building. International work in this now direction presupposes the involvement of other key international organizations in this area. As a first step, the WHO Executive Board will discuss the content of a WHO report covering this subject in January 2003. It is hoped that this report could form the basis for a future initiative towards a systematic, coordinated, multi-organizational and international evaluation of certain GM foods

Ok that was 1990 to 2000 with the world health organization and others. But the questions and answers were what was asked and answered at that time. Read on this is now 2016 and this is the new release and it's very different from what you have just read. It takes time to see what crap is in the crops that we the human race are being told is ok, we eat it they don't we get sick they don't.

This is not a work of fiction; this is based on real people I have taken the names of the parties involved out to protect their identities.

The truth about GMOs

This report is from March 2015; the world health organization (WHO) concluded that glyphosate, the herbicide weed-killer, is probably carcinogenic to humans. Glyphosate is by far the most widely used herbicide because it is the weed-killer that genetically modified corn and soybeans are engineered to "tolerate" with GM varieties now accounting for 90 percent or more of the market for corn and soybeans, glyphosate is being liberally sprayed over ever-more-vast tracts of farmland with farmers secure in the knowledge that their crops won't be harmed by the herbicide.

Apparently humans may not be so tolerant, and animals in feeding trials

certainly aren't. One study in community residents reported increases in blood markers of chromosomal damage (micronuclei) after glyphosate formulations were sprayed nearby." Because there have been no long-term human feeding trials, the evidence is limited, mainly to studies of agricultural exposures. Human feeding trials are considered unethical, so the gold standard for epidemiological research is the animal study. WHO found, in its year- long expert scientific review of the evidence from government and peer reviewed studies, that "there is convincing evidence that glyphosate also can cause cancer in laboratory animals." That finding makes glyphosate a "probable carcinogen" for humans, according to accepted WHO standards. That probably will not quiet the consensus campaigners, but it should. A peer – reviewed study of the research found that about half of the animal-feeding studies conducted in recent years found cause for concern. The other half did not and as the researchers noted, "most of these studies have been conducted by biotechnology companies responsible for commercializing these GM plants."

The only consensus that GM food is safe is among industry-funded researchers.

Product placement for GMOs; call it product placement, like the nearly subliminal advertising technique in which soda makers pay a movie producer to have the characters all drink there soda. Biotechnology companies and their powerful advocates are succeeding in a well- placed campaign to get GM safety declared "settled science." The article hardly touches the GM controversy or the science. It focuses on the interesting and important question of how people, including scientists, interpret scientific evidence in a way tainted by confirmation bias, the tendency to more readily believe evidence that confirms one's existing beliefs. We are asked to accept, that it is safe to eat food containing genetically modified organisms because, the experts point out, there is no evidence that it isn't and no reason to believe that altering genes precisely in a lab is more dangerous than altering them wholesale through traditional breeding. What we are seeing is a concerted campaign to do exactly what Nation Geographic has knowing or unknowingly done: paint GMO critics as anti-science while offering no serious discussion of the scientific controversy that still rages.

The consensus on the safety of GM food is perfectly clear: there is no consensus. That's what the independent peer-reviewed literature says. And that's what the National Geographic's exhibit on food series, in its Washington headquarters, says the "long term health and ecological consequences are unknown." And that is an accurate statement of the consensus, or the lack of it.

The debate is over what level of precaution should apply before allowing the large-scale commercialization of this new technology, and anyone stating that there is a scientific consensus on GM safety is coming down squarely against precaution. Reasonable people disagree, and that does not make them "science doubters".

According to the Department of Agriculture, 90 percent of the corn and cotton and 93 percent of the soybeans planted in the last year were genetically modified.

These are commodity crops mostly for animal feed and fuel ethanol, but they also provide the corn syrup in bottled beverages and the soy lecithin in chocolate bars, and with the public still leery of the technology, it was perhaps inevitable that after a stretch of relative quiet the GMO wars would heat up again.

The latest front is over food labeling: in the past two years, ballot initiatives that would have mandated labeling narrowly lost in Washington State and California: while the debate about the impact of GM crops on the environment continues, the question of their effect on human health looks increasingly settled. The National Academy of Sciences, the American Medical Association, the World Health Organization, Britain's Royal Society, The European Commission, and the American Association for the Advancement of Science, among others, have all surveyed the substantial research literature and found no evidence that the GM foods on the market today are unsafe to eat.

Much of its 1.5 billion research budget goes into traditional plant breeding; the same craft the botanist Gregor Mendel pioneered on his pea plants a century and a half ago, though at a scale and speed that would boggle the friar's mind.

This company is also researching the targeted use of bacteria, fungi and other living organisms to protect and nourish seeds: farming technologies that borrow, at least conceptually, from organic agriculture. In perhaps the biggest shift, they are moving into computing.

Through the purchase of two companies they have begun offering software and hardware products that gather and process information relevant to a farmer--- data about temperature, rain, soil, seeds, and pests. Big Data has already transformed everything from retail logistics to dating; they believe it can do the same for farming

The European food safety authority has discovered a hidden gene in 54 of 84 commercially approved genetically engineered crops, a finding that highlights deep flaws in the regulatory process. Plant pathologists speak out about the potential dangers of the viral gene fragment in GE plants, stating it may confer "significant potential for harm" and call for a total recall of affected crops.

Plants expressing the viral gene fragment exhibit gene expression abnormalities, which indicate that the protein produced by gene functions as a toxin. The known targets of its activity are also found in human cells, so there is potential for this plant toxin to also have toxic effects on humans.

At present the only way to avoid GE foods is to eliminate processed foods from your grocery list, and buy primarily whole foods grown according to organic standards. The need for labeling of GE foods is also becoming more apparent in order to allow for health monitoring. The potential dangers of genetically engineered foods is that such crops might have wholly unforeseen consequences. In recent years, such suspicions have increasingly proven correct, and now researchers have released another bombshell.

Genetic manipulation of crops, and more recently food animals, is a dangerous game that has repeatedly revealed that assumptions about how genetic alterations work and the effects it has on animals and humans who consume such foods, are deeply flawed and incomplete.

No-one knows, what quantity, location or timing of protein production would be of significance for assessment, and so answers necessary to perform science – based risk assessment are unlikely to emerge soon. It is perhaps the most basic assumption in all of risk assessment that the developer of a new product provides regulators with accurate information about what is being assessed. Perhaps the next most basic assumption is that regulators independently verify this information.

The FDA cleared the way for GE (Genetically Engineered) Atlantic salmon to be farmed for human consumption. Thanks to added language in the federal spending bill, the product will require special labeling so at least consumers will have the ability to identify the GE salmon in stores. However, it's imperative all GE foods be labeled, which is currently still being denied.

The biotech industry is trying to push the QR code as an answer for consumer concerns about GE foods. QR stands for Quick Response, and the code can be scanned and read by smart phones and other QR readers.

The code brings you to a product website that provides further details about the product. There's nothing forcing companies to declare GMOs on their website. On the contrary, GE foods are allowed to be promoted as "natural" which further adds to the confusion. These so-called "smart labels" hardly improve access to information. Instead by making finding the truth time- consuming and cumbersome, food makers can be assured that most people will remain ignorant about the presence of GMOs in their products. Besides everyone has a right to know what is in the food you are eating! You shouldn't have to own a smartphone to obtain this information.

The way GMOs have been creepily introduced into our food chain is quite baffling. I mean, you would think that integrating a foreign body into our food without having carried out the most reasonably extensive studies common sense can buy would raise at least a little concern from our government. Many countries of the European Union are GMO free zones. Remember, when talking about GMOs, we are not talking about the food old selection techniques that saved us from starvation and allowed us to march on the evolution path. In a sensible world, even dreaming of playing God with the most essential elements of our human survival would result in a generous backhand in hopes of snatching the delusional dreamer out of his daze. But sadly, the truth is that we are actually living this nightmare, where bad turns to worse, and where our cherished memories of a government willing to go to bat for us gets blurrier by the minute. So we ask, how did our government allow us to become the mice of these experiments it seems pressed to conduct on the wider population? But wait, this is unfair. Why should our government bear the brunt of the blame? Our government is equipped with strict safety assessment mechanisms, ensuring that all novel food products are scientifically scrutinized by Health Canada. Excellent point! These novel products do have to be evaluated by a process that lasts between seven and ten years, which sees them, put through a battery of tests. How could I forget this bulletproof mechanism? Crisis averted! Well there is just a small detail that might be worth mentioning here. Enter: SmartStax. This GM corn was approved by Health Canada in 2009 without any testing, even though it had never been introduced in our food chain. Why? Because it's eight distinct genetically modified traits (six of which each release their own insecticidal toxin while the remaining two resist a couple of herbicides) had already been evaluated, independently and were deemed harmless. So Health Canada didn't recognize SmartStax as a new product necessitating the aforementioned scrutiny, and this despite the fact that it was the first time all of its GM components were expressed in a single plant. Seriously what are we left with when the precautionary measures adopted by our government are simply too weak. We are left with a chilling study that confirms our inner voice's long repeated warning "food should not be grown in labs.

Chemical additives in your food: we don't just want our food to taste good; it also has to look good. As a result, food producers use any of 14,000 laboratory-made additives to make our food appear fresher, more attractive or last longer on the shelf. The longer manufacturers use these additives, the more we learn about their impacts. While some additives are harmless, others cause everything from hives and asthma to nausea and headaches in some people. Some experts recommend avoiding foods listing more than five or six ingredients or ingredients of longer than three syllables and purchase foods that contain such natural additives as fruits and vegetables.

15 chemical additives and their possible side effects will help you to decipher ingredients at your supermarket.

METHYLCYCLOPROPENE

This gas is pumped into creates of apples to stop them from producing ethylene, the natural hormone that ripens fruit. Commonly known as Smart-Fresh, this chemical preserves apples for up to a year and bananas up to a month. Sulphur dioxide serves the same purpose when sprayed on grapes.

ARTIFICIAL COLOURS

Researchers in the early 1900s developed many artificial colors from coal-tar dyes and petrochemicals. Over the years, the FDA banned many of these chemicals as proven carcinogens (cancer-exacerbating agents). Today the FDA only allows 10 colors in foods four of which are restricted to specific uses. The restriction suggests some risks remain.

ARTIFICIAL FLAVORING

This blanket term refers to hundreds of laboratory chemicals designed to mimic natural flavors. For example, some imitation vanilla flavorings are made from petroleum or paper-mill waste. In fact, a single artificial flavoring can be created from hundreds of individual chemicals. New studies suggest artificial flavoring additives can cause changes in behavior.

ASPARTAME

This sugar substitute is sold commercially as Equal and Nutra-Sweet and was hailed as a savior for dieters unhappy with saccharine's unpleasant after –taste. Unfortunately one out of 20,000 babies is born without the ability to metabolize phenylalanine, one of the two amino acids in aspartame. As a result, it's not recommended for pregnant women or infants.

ASTAXANTHIN

Almost 90-percent of salmon sold in supermarkets today come from farms. The diet of farmed salmon doesn't include crustaceans, which contains a natural astaxanthin that causes pink flesh in wild salmon. As a result, producers add astaxanthin to farm – salmon diets for that fresh –from –the –water appearance. Astaxanthin is manufactured from coal tar.

BENZOIC ACID/SODIUM NENZOATE

Often added to milk and meat products, these preservatives are used in many foods, including drinks, low-sugar products, cereals and meats. Both temporarily inhibit the proper functioning of digestive enzymes and cause headaches, stomach upset, asthma attacks and hyperactivity in children.

BHA (BUTYLATED HYDROXYANISOLE) AND BHT (BUTYLATED HYDROXYTOLUENE)

These antioxidants are similar but non-identical petroleum- derived chemicals add to oil- containing foods as a preservative and to delay rancidity. They are most commonly found in crackers, cereals, sausages, dried meats and other foods with added fats. The World Health Organization's International Agency for Research on Cancer considers BHA a possible human carcinogen.

CANTHAXANTHIN

Egg yolks don't always come out golden yellow, so producers use this pigment to make them more palatable. Although the amounts used are very small, tests have shown greater quantities of canthaxanthin can cause retinal damage.

EMULSIFIERS

Emulsifiers, made from vegetable fats, glycerol and organic acids, extend the shelf life of bread products and allow liquids that wouldn't normally mix, such as oil and water, to combine smoothly. Many reduced-fat or low-calorie products use emulsifiers. Commercial emulsifiers also are used in low – calorie butter, margarine, salad dressings, mayonnaise and ice cream. Emulsifying agents used in foods include agar, albumin, alginates, casein, egg yolk, glycerol monostearate, xanthan gums, Irish moss, lecithin and soaps.

HIGH-FRUCTOSE CORN SYRUP

This ubiquitous sweetener helps maintain moisture while preserving freshness. A little fructose isn't a problem but the sheer quantity of "hidden" fructose in processed foods is startling. The consumption of large quantities has been fingered as a causative factor in heart disease. It raises blood levels of cholesterol and triglyceride fats, while making blood cells more prone to clotting and accelerating the aging process.

MONOSODIUM GLUTAMATE (MSG)

There was much hue and cry years ago when the public learned Chinese restaurants commonly add MSG to Chinese foods as a flavor enhancer. We then learned MSG could be found in many other processed products. Such as: salad dressings, condiments, seasonings, bouillons and snack chips. Some reports indicate MSG causes tightening in the chest, headaches and a burning sensation in the neck and forearms. While MSG is made of components found in our bodies- water, sodium and glutamate (a common amino acid) ingesting it is an entirely different matter.

OLESTRA

The FDA approved this fake fat for use in snack foods several years ago, over objections from dozens of researchers. Their concern was that Olestra inhibits our ability to absorb the healthy vitamins in fruits and vegetables thought to reduce the risk of cancer and heart disease. Even at low doses, Olestra is commonly known to cause "anal leakage" and other gastrointestinal problems. Perhaps this is why the FDA requires foods containing Olestra carry a warning label.

PARTIALLY-HYDROGENATED OILS

Hydrogenation is the process of heating oil and passing hydrogen bubbles through it. The fatty acids in the oil then acquire some of the hydrogen, which makes it denser. If you fully hydrogenate, you create a solid (a fat) out of the oil. But if you stop part way, you create semi-solid, partially hydrogenated oil with the consistency of butter. Because this process is so much cheaper than using butter, partially –hydrogenated oils are found in many, many foods. Their addictive properties have linked partially-hydrogenated oils to weight problems caused by a slowed metabolism and the development of diabetes, cancer and heart disease.

POTASSIUM BROMATE

Potassium bromate increases volume in white flour, breads and rolls. Most bromate rapidly breaks down to an innocuous form, but it is known to cause cancer in animals- and even small amounts in bread can create a risk for humans. California requires a cancer warning on the product label if potassium bromate is an ingredient.

SODIUM NITRITE AND NITRATE

These closely related chemicals have been used for centuries to preserve meat. While nitrate itself is harmless, it easily converts to nitrite which, when combined with secondary-amines compounds form nitrosamines, a powerful cancer-exacerbating chemical. This chemical reaction occurs easily during the frying process.

HOW FOOD AFFECTS YOUR BEHAVIOR

Food additives and poor diet could help explain poor school performance, criminal behavior, alcoholism and the growing numbers of Alzheimer's patients. High sugar content and starchy carbohydrates lead to excessive insulin release, which in turn leads to falling blood sugar levels, or hypoglycemia. Hypoglycemia causes the brain to secrete glutamate in levels that can cause agitation, depression, anger, anxiety, panic attacks and an increase in suicide risk. The glutamate that causes this is identical to the flavor-enhancing monosodium glutamate (MSG) and its chemical cousins, which are found in thousands of food products, further exacerbating the problem. Repeated hypoglycemic episodes increase the risk of neurodegenerative diseases, such as Alzheimer's disease, Parkinson's and ALS (Lou Gehrig's). In children, hypoglycemia often leads to hyperactivity. In both children and adults, it can cause violent and aggressive behavior. In older people, there can be mental confusion.

An anti – hypoglycemic diet would consist of lean meat and lots of fresh vegetables. Another key is limiting sugars and starches.

Canadians and Americans spend about 90percent of their food budget on processed foods, which contain a staggering number of artificial food additives, preservatives, colors and flavor enhancers. It is virtually impossible to identify them all and what is their true impact on your health. However, some we know more about than others. For example, there's a substantial body of evidence backing up the claim that sugar, artificial sweeteners and MSG have a radically negative impact on your body. Other hazardous food additives that should be avoided, such as:

Sodium nitrate, sodium benzoate, BHA and BHT, propyl gall ate, trans-fats, Acesulfame-K, food dyes, olestra, potassium bromate.

The issue of whether or not food additives such as artificial colors contribute to behavioral problems in children has been disputed for many years. However, the tide is finally turning. A carefully designed, randomized, double –blind, placebo-controlled study in the journal the lancet last year concluded that a variety of common food dyes, and the preservative sodium benzoate found in many soft drinks, fruit juices and salad dressings-do cause some children to become more hyperactive and distractible. The study also found that the E-numbered food dyes do as much damage to children's brains as leak in gasoline, resulting in a significant reduction in IQ. The results of this study have prompted the British Food Standards Agency (FSA) to issue an immediate advisory to parents, warning them to limit their children's intake of additives if they notice an effect on behavior. They're also advising the food industry to voluntarily remove the six food dyes named in the study, and replace them with natural alternatives if possible. The U.S., however, has not followed suit in issuing any similar warnings to American parents.

Beware of banned food additives in children's medicines too!

Another thing you need to be aware of, as a parent, is that when an ingredient is banned for use in food, it is not automatically banned for use in other areas such as medicine. According to an expose' by the British Food Commission, food additives that have already been banned for use in food and beverages are still used in a majority of pediatric over –the – counter medicines. The survey found that all but one medicine out of 41 contained an additive that had been banned. The additives found in these drugs included: Synthetic (azo dyes) Maltitol and sorbitol, Benzoate and sulphite preservatives, and chloroform. This is just one more reason why it is so important to question what your doctor or any other health professional may prescribe or recommend for your child, no matter what side of the counter it comes from, as many pediatric drugs can certainly be harmful, if not downright toxic to your child's health.

Another study that measured the visible effects of sugar consumptions gave children the amount of sugar equal to one soda. As a result, their test scores went down, in fact, one hour after consuming the sugar they made twice as many mistakes. The sugar –loaded students also showed more "inappropriate behavior" during free play. Sugar has a profound influence on your brain function, and your psychological function. When you consume excess amounts of sugar, your body releases excess amounts of insulin, which in turn causes a drop in your blood sugar, also known as hypoglycemia. Hypoglycemia in turn causes your brain to secrete glutamate. Which is a "Messenger molecule" that serves an important function in your body; however, when excess amounts of glutamate are excreted it can wreak havoc with your brain and nervous system, causing a variety of side effects such as agitation, depression, anger, anxiety and panic attacks. The glutamate produced in your body is identical to the flavor-enhancing monosodium glutamate (MSG), which is added to thousands of food products that boost your body's glutamate load even higher. MSG is used in countless foods in your supermarket, local restaurants, school cafeterias and more. Everything from soup to crackers to meats may contain it because MSG, as dangerous as it is, makes food taste good and it is dirt cheap just like sugar. There are a couple of main reasons why MSG is one of the worst food additives on the market. First as Dr. Blaylock explains in his book Excitotoxins: the taste that kills, MSG is an excitotoxin, which means that it acts as a poison that overexcites your cells to the point of serious damage. MSG is non – discriminatory in its destructive path and can cause serious side effects throughout your bodily systems, including: cardiac, circulatory, gastrointestinal, muscular, neurological, visual, respiratory, urological/genital and skin. Other studies have confirmed that early exposure to MSG and other Excitotoxins can destroy neurons in a crucial part of your brain, which can lead to gross obesity.MSG can be hidden in food labels, under names like broth, casein, hydrolyzed, autolyzed, natural flavors, and more, making it extremely difficult to identify.

Incredibly, even infant formulas and baby food contains this poison, even though babies and infants, who are four times more sensitive than adults to the toxic effects of this chemical, are the most at risk. In the 1970s food processors "voluntarily" took processed free glutamic acid (MSG) out of baby food. That didn't mean it was entirely removed. It was merely hidden deeper. A 1995 review of MSG toxicity by the Federation of American Societies for Experimental Biology (FASEB) concluded that infant formula contained a dose of glutamate (the toxic ingredient in MSG) in the form of caseinate (cow's milk protein) that can produce the very same brain injury seen in experimental animals. MSG also finds its way into baby food in the form of fertilizers called Omega Protein Refined/ Hydrolyzed Fish Emulsion or "Steam Hydrolyzed Feather Meal," both of which contain hydrolyzed proteins.

The use of MSG in food manufacturing and processing is so pervasive, they've even found a way to use it on fresh produce. A product called AuxiGro WP Plant Metabolic Primer (auxigro), produced by Bio Agriculture contains both hydrolyzed proteins and about 29 percent monosodium glutamate. Auxigro is used as a desiccant, disinfectant, fertilizer, fungicide, and growth regulator to increase yield and prevent powdery mildew in various crops, it's a "Metabolic Primer" that increases plant productivity by priming plant metabolic pathways associated with growth, plant disease resistance, flowering, and "quality characteristics" of the produce. Despite searching for information on this product; it proved to be profoundly aggravating, as virtually all official links related to it were mysteriously broken, however, it wasn't entirely fruitless, AuxiGro has been sprayed on fruits, vegetables and nuts for a long time along with; celery, fresh market cucumbers, edible navy and pinto beans, grapes, bulb onions, bell, green and jalapeno peppers, iceberg head lettuce, romaine and butter leaf lettuce, peanuts, potatoes, snap beans, strawberries, processing tomatoes, and watermelons, as of 2000 auxigro was registered for use in California on tomatoes, almonds, apricots, cherries, plums, nectarines, peaches, prunes, grapes, (includes grapes to be used in wine), and onions.

And in 2004 they requested approval to add crops (including broccoli, Brussel sprouts, cabbage, cauliflower, kale, collards, turnips, rutabaga, mustard, watercress, and kohlrabi) to the list of crops approved for auxigro use. Today there is no known commercial crop that has not been approved for treatment with MSG by the U.S. Environmental Protection Agency (EPA). Bio Agriculture has also requested approval to use Auxigro on Organic Crops, in all states. It does not appear as though their request for use on organic crops has ever been approved, per se. however, MSG –containing ingredients are not specified on the National Organic Program's list of prohibited substances either, so it's difficult to discern whether or not it's being used in some organic farming as well. My advice is you find a butcher's shop for your meat make sure it is antibiotic free, grow your own vegetables or buy them locally grown, lots of people selling from their homes, buy your eggs from free range chickens. This can take some time out of your day, but it is worth it believe me remember you cannot buy good health; and you are what you eat. If we do not start now we never will; it is time we took control of what and how we eat. You are not only doing this for you but also for generations yet to come. Think about it.

Food labeling tricks the industry hopes you never learn

What is the first thing you need to know about reading food labels; too often, people with the best of intentions don't realize that unless you read the entire label, you're not going to get a true idea of the food's ingredients. Even then, you have to know how to interpret what the label says to be absolutely certain that you are getting what you want.

I'm going to help you with that

The best advice is to simply not eat any processed foods at all. But if you must, here is a short list of ingredients and phrases to avoid- artificial colors, artificial flavorings, artificial sweeteners, high fructose corn syrup, sodium nitrates or nitrites. Maybe you didn't have the ingredient list on you "natural" product until you got home, only to notice some very un-natural looking ingredients listed there, and wondered how there could be such an enormous difference between the front of the bag and the back. Most of what is on the label is marketing hype and splashy design work, made only to seduce you into believing the product is good for you, you have to be very market –savvy to find the truth, because labels have fooled even the smartest shoppers, it's easy to be duped, if you don't know what to look for. Have you ever wondered how many people actually select their food based on what the label says? In 2006 a survey was taken on more than a 1,000 adults. The results might surprise you. 80 percent read labels for things like calories, fat, sugar, and salt, but 44 percent buy food products, regardless of what the food label says. 65 percent of women read labels, compared to 51 percent of men. 39 percent of young people ages 18 to 29 said they look at calories on food labels, but 60 percent of them buy them, regardless of the label.

You might be surprised to learn that the FDA does not require foods to be laboratory tested for nutritional content. While the FDA does check food labels, they only check to see whether or not the nutrition facts panel is present- not whether or not it's accurate.

The labeling law allows food companies to simple estimate average values for fat, protein, carbohydrates, and sugar; for any given product based on a standard list of ingredients. So, how accurate do they have to be to avoid violating labeling laws? The FDA says a 20 percent margin of error is acceptable. Even getting 20 percent more of fat or sugar than you want will really add up over time. But the truth is, it much worse than that.

You can expect labels to lie! The FDA estimates that roughly ten percent of food product labels contain inaccuracies. Ten percent; really, when actually analyzed by a laboratory, most grocery and restaurant foods are much higher than advertised in fats, carbohydrates, sugars and sodium. According to a BBC news article, food testers analyzed 570 nutrients listed on 70 products. Only 7 percent matched what the label said- levels of fat, salt, calories and carbs were inaccurate in 93 percent of products were surprising: one biscuit or cookie was found to have three times the amount of saturated fat claimed on the label, one type of pizza was found to have 80 percent more fat, Cadbury's light truffles were found to have 23 percent more fat than was claimed on the label. A 2008 report by the Government Accountability Office found that about 24 percent of food labels were inaccurate. Also in 2008 Good Morning America hired a lab to test a dozen packaged food products to see if the nutrients matched the labels, and all 12 products exceeded what was claimed on the label, in one way or another primarily fat, sugar, and sodium. Manufacturers get away with this because punishment for violations is a joke, for a first offence, information about the food is entered into a database, but the product is still allowed on store shelves. If a second violation is detected within 60 days, then the product may be suspended. But here is the catch: since food testing is very infrequent, it is highly unlikely that a second offence will be caught within their 60-day time frame. This effectively allows food manufactures to do whatever they want and slant their claims however they wish, based on the demographic they want to manipulate. The marketing of children's foods is a perfect example.

Prevention institute investigated package labeling for children's food in 2010. They found 84 percent of products advertised as "healthiest picks for kids" did not meet even basic nutritional standards; and the next time you see “”zero trans fats” on a label, don’t believe it. Manufactures are allowed to use that phrase as long as the product contains less than 0.5 grams per serving. Look at the ingredients list and see if it contains some hydrogenated or partially hydrogenated oils.

There are a few buzzwords to watch out for on the front of the box that says absolutely nothing about the true nutritional value of what’s inside; line = all natural ingredients, or 100 percent natural, no artificial preservatives (do they mean they only use real preservatives?),

Real fruit, (just because the package shows a picture of an apple doesn’t mean the apple has to be in there). Statements like those are unregulated and are designed to appeal to the gullible health- conscious, but do not reflect nutritional content. Marketers hope you are uninformed enough to accept those statements at face value- hoping you will just grab the bag and go. Even phrases like “all organic” have little meaning without the official USCD Organic seal, which is your best assurance of quality.

Growers and manufactures of organic products bearing the USDA seal have to meet the strictest standards of any of the currently available organic labels, in terms of being free of antibiotics and growth hormones, pesticides, heavy metals, preservatives, chemicals, irradiation etc. that said, even the USDA organic seal has been greatly compromised over the past several years.

Organic food now represents a $16-billion business, with sales growing by as much as 20 percent per year. Unfortunately the quality and meaning of the organic label is undergoing an equally fast decline. Organic foods were once truly raised naturally, on small farms with great integrity, but with skyrocketing popularity of the organic food industry, big business has now stepped in and tainted many of the principles upon which the organic label was founded. A well-known mega store for instance, is now the largest organic retailer in the United States. According to the organic consumers association, the mega – store is: selling organic milk that comes from intensive confinement factory farm dairies, importing cheap organic foods and ingredients from China and Brazil, posting signs in its stores that mislead people into believing that non-organic items are actually organic.

The sad fact is; you are being ripped off by much of the organic food you are buying. For example, consider all of those “ORGANIC” junk foods like ice cream, crackers, cookies, pizza, and potato chips. A potato chip is one of the worst foods you can eat, regardless of whether or not the potato is organic. Yet big business is cashing in on your desire to "have your cake and it too" by trying to make you believe you can eat cake, cookies, ice cream and potato chips without feeling guilty; because they are organic.

The same deception is beginning to happen with the word "local". How local is local? Is it grown within your City, Province, or Country? "Local" is yet another unregulated term that clever marketers are using to increase sales. Without visiting the farm, it is hard to know what "local" really is.

Additives that should not be in our food; in 1958, Congressman James Delaney of New York authored an amendment to the Food, Drugs and Cosmetics Act of 1938 called the Delaney Clause. Stating:

"The secretary of the food and drug administration shall not approve for use in food any chemical additive found to induce cancer in man, or after tests, found to induce cancer in animals."

The problem is, additives that were "GRAS" (generally regarded as safe) prior to this amendment were "grandfathered in"- and some of them are now known to be carcinogenic. The following are a few examples of food additives to watch out for in your ingredient list:

MSG- a flavor enhancer, this agent is a potent neurotoxin that can cause anything from migraines to Parkinson's or Alzheimer's disease; hidden in a multitude of other ingredients, including autolyzed yeast, glutamate, textured protein, gelatin, natural flavors, barley malt and soy sauce, etc.

Sodium nitrite and nitrate – preservatives added to processed meats that are carcinogenic.

BHA AND BHT – preservatives added to processed foods, also linked to cancer.

Potassium bromate – added to many white flours and baked goods, this endocrine disruptor damages your thyroid and can cause psychiatric and cardiac problems; most countries have banned it.

Common food dyes – such as citrus red No 2, which is used to dye your oranges orange; unless you buy organic oranges. Like most FD& C dyes, this dye is derived from coal tar, which is a human carcinogen. If you zest a non-organic orange, you may be consuming this dye.

Until we succeed in getting a labeling law for all genetically modified foods, the only way to be somewhat assured a food is non-GMO is if it is labeled specifically as such, or if it holds the official USDA organic seal; and even this is no longer a certainty due to widespread seed contamination. Your chance of acquiring a genetically modified Hawaiian papaya is 50/50 – even if you're buying one that's certified organic.

The idea that you can identify GM produce by its PLU code is a myth. There are no easy answers when it comes to deciphering food labels, but there are simple strategies that can help ensure you know exactly what you and your family are eating: = avoid packaged or processed foods, select whole foods, shopping around the perimeter of the grocery store, preparing your food at home.

It really comes down to a change in mindset- choosing to eat "real" food that has been minimally processed and tampered with- like fresh produce, organic meat and eggs. Even better choose food that is humanely and sustainably raised /produced near you. Shop at your local farmers market or coop; get to know your farmers personally.

What you need to know about GMOs

Genetically modified organisms or genetically engineered goods, are live organisms whose genetic components have been artificially manipulated in a laboratory setting; through creating unstable combinations of plant, animal, bacteria, and even viral genes that do not occur in nature or through traditional crossbreeding methods.

You need to contact your MP or senators, ask them to oppose any compromise that would block or delay labeling laws. You are not doing this for yourself but for your children and their children.

POTENTIAL HEALTH HAZARDS: OF GENETICALLY ENGINEETED FOODS.

This article discusses the potential health risks of genetically engineered foods (GMOs). It draws on some of what you have already read but it does bear repeating. It also sights three notable books and highlights one in particular. Jeffery Smith's Genetic Roulette: The documented health risks of genetically engineered foods.

Genetically engineered foods saturate our diet today. In the US alone, over 80% of all processed foods contain them. Others include grains like rice, corn and wheat; legumes like soybeans and soy products; vegetable oils, soft drinks, salad dressings, vegetables and fruits; dairy products including eggs, meat, chicken, pork and other animal products; and even infant formula plus a vast array of hidden additives and ingredients in processed foods (like in tomato sauce, ice cream, margarine and peanut butter). Consumers don't know what they are eating because labeling is prohibited, yet the danger is clear.

Independently conducted studies show the more of these foods we eat, the greater the potential harm to our health.

I personally have been researching GMO for over twenty years.

Today consumers are kept in the dark and are part of an uncontrolled unregulated mass human experiment the results of which are unknown. Yet the risks are enormous, it will take years to learn them, and when we finally know it will be too late to reverse the damage if it is proven conclusively that genetically engineered foods harm human health as growing numbers of independent experts believe.

When given a choice, animals avoid GM foods. This was learned by observing a flock of geese that annually visit an Illinois pond and feed on soybeans from an adjacent farm. After half the acreage had GM crops, the geese ate only from the non- GMO side. Another observation showed 40 deer ate organic soybeans from one field but shunned the GMO kind across the road. The same thing happened with GM corn. Potential harm to adults is magnified for children.

Unchecked and unregulated, human health and safety are at risk because once GMOs enter the food chain, the genie is out of the bottle for keeps. Thankfully, resistance is growing worldwide, many millions are opposed, but reversing the tide will not be easy.

I'm hopeful that people will prevail over profits. Hopefully I'm right because human health and safety must never be compromised. Resistance already halted the introduction of new crop varieties, and i believe with enough momentum existing ones may end up withdrawn.

A pew survey reported that 29% of Americans, representing 87 million people, strongly oppose these foods and believe they are unsafe. That's a respectable start if backed up with efforts to avoid them. Smyth founded Responsible Technology. Org in 2003 to promote the responsible use of technology and stop GM foods and crops through both grassroots and national strategies; it seeks safe alternatives and aims to ban the genetic engineering of our food supply and all outdoor releases of (GM) organisms, at least until (or unless scientific opinion) believes such products are safe and appropriate based on independent and reliable data. IRT urges consumers to become educated about the risks, mobilize to combat them and act in our mutual self-interest. It's beginning to happen, and I believe there is an excellent chance that food manufactures will abandon GM foods in the near future "if a public groundswell demands it". Although GMOs present one of the greatest dangers, with informed motivated people; it is one of the easiest global issues to solve.

I really hope this information helps and answers some of your questions on this. All the information on this is research I have done over many years in order to educate myself; so I could help my clients with their fears and concerns. I decided to put it in this book, because I believe you should know and decide for yourself. All the information in here you can find for yourself all you have to do is look.

I think it's time you did that for yourself as well as your family.

MENTAL ILLNESS AND ADDICTIONS

The terms "mental illness" and "addiction" refer to a wide range of disorders that affect mood, thinking and behaviour. Examples include depression, anxiety disorders, schizophrenia as well as substance use disorders and problems gambling. Mental illness and addictions can be associated with distress and /or impairment of functioning. Symptoms vary from mild to severe. In any given year 1 in 5 Canadians experiences a mental health or addiction problem. 70% of mental health problems have their onset during childhood or adolescence. Young people aged 15 to 24 are more likely to experience mental illness and /or substance use disorders than any other age group. Men have higher rates of addiction than women, while women have higher rates of mood and anxiety disorders. People with a mental illness are twice as likely to have a substance use problem compared to the general population. At least 20% of people with a mental illness have a co-occurring substance use problem. For people with schizophrenia, the number may be as high as 50%. Similarly, people with substance use problems are up to 3 times more likely to have a mental illness. More than 15% of people with a substance use problem have a co-occurring mental illness. Canadians in the lowest income group are 3 to 4 times more likely than those in the highest income group to report poor to fair mental health. Studies in various Canadian cities indicate that between 23% and 67% of homeless people report having a mental illness. Mental illness is a leading cause of disability in Canada. People with mental illness and addictions are more likely to die prematurely than the general population. Mental illness can cut 10 to 20 years of a person's life expectancy. The disease burden of mental illness and addiction in Ontario is 1.5 times higher than all cancers put together and more than 7 times that of all infectious diseases. This includes years lived with less than full function and years lost to early death. Tobacco, the most widely used addictive substance, is the leading cause of premature mortality in Canada. Evidence suggests that smoking is responsible for nearly 17% of all deaths. Among Ontarians aged 25 to 34, 1 of every 8 deaths is related to opioid use.

Nearly 4,000 Canadians die by suicide each year and average of almost 11 suicides a day. It affects people of all ages and backgrounds. About 230,000 Ontarians over 18, or 2.2% of the adult population, report having seriously contemplated suicide in the past year. More than 75% of suicides involve men, but women attempt suicide 3 to 4 times more often. In 2012 suicide accounted for 17% of deaths among aged 10 to 14, 28% among youth aged 15 to 19 and 25% among young adults aged 20 to 24. After accidents it is the second leading cause of death for people aged 15 to 34. More than half of suicides involve people aged 45 or older. First Nations youth die by suicide about 5 to 6 times more often than non –Aboriginal youth. Suicide rates for Inuit youth are among the highest in the world, at 11 times the national average. A survey taken in 2008 says just 50% of Canadians would tell friends or co- workers that they have a family member with a mental illness, compared to 72% who would discuss a diagnosis of cancer and 68% who would talk about a family member having diabetes. 42% of Canadians were unsure whether they would socialize with a friend who has a mental illness. 55% of Canadians said they would be unlikely to enter a spousal relationship with someone who has a mental illness. 46% of Canadians thought people use the term mental illness as an excuse for bad behaviour, and 27% said they would be fearful of being around someone who suffers from serious mental illness. In 2015: 57% believed that the stigma associated with mental illness has been reduced compared to 5 years ago. 81% are now more aware of mental health issues compared to 5 years ago. 70% believe attitudes about mental health issues have changed for the better compared to 5 years ago. But stigma remains: 64% of Ontario workers would be concerned about how work would be affected if a colleague had a mental illness. 39% of Ontario workers indicate that they would not tell their managers if they were experiencing a mental health problem. While mental illness accounts for about 10% of the burden of disease in Ontario, it receives just 7% of health care dollars. Relative to this burden, mental health is Ontario is underfunded by about 1.5 billion. The mental health strategy for Canada recommends raising the proportion of health spending that is devoted to mental health to 9% by 2022. 17% of Canadians aged 15 or older report having a mental health care need in the past year: one third of those individuals report that their needs were not fully met. The rate is even higher in children and youth. In 2013-2014, 5% of ED visits and 18% of inpatient hospitalizations for children and youth age 5 to 24 in Canada were for a mental disorder. Individuals with a mental illness are much less likely to be employed. Unemployment rates are as high as 70% to 90% for people with the most severe mental illnesses. In any given week at least 500,000 employed Canadians are unable to work due to mental health problems. This includes approximately 355,000 disability cases due to mental or behavioural disorders, plus approximately 175,000 full-time workers absent from work due to mental illness. The economic burden of mental illness in Canada is estimated at $51 billion per year. This includes health care costs, lost productivity, and reductions in health – related quality of life.

UNDERSTANDING DRUG ABUSE AND ADDICTION: Many people do not understand why or how other people become addicted to drugs. It is often mistakenly assumed that drug abusers lack moral principles or willpower and that they could stop using simply by choosing to change their behaviour. In reality, drug addiction is a complex disease, and quitting takes more than good intentions or a strong will. In fact, because drugs change the brain in ways that foster compulsive drug abuse, quitting is difficult, even for those who are ready to do so. Through scientific advances, we know more about how drugs work in the brain than ever, and we also know that drug addiction can be successfully treated to help people stop abusing and lead productive lives. Drug abuse and addiction have negative consequences for individuals and for society. Estimates of the total overall cost of substance abuse in the United States, including productivity and health- and crime-related costs, exceed $600 billion annually. This includes approximately $193 billion for illicit drugs, $193 billion for tobacco, and $235 billion for alcohol. As staggering as these numbers are, they do not fully describe the breadth of destructive public health and safety implications of drug abuse and addiction, such as family disintegration, loss of employment, failure in school, domestic violence and child abuse.

Addiction is a chronic, often relapsing brain disease that causes compulsive drug seeking and use, despite harmful consequences to the addicted individual and to those around him or her. Although the initial decision to take drugs is voluntary for most people, the brain changes that occur over time challenge an addicted person's self-control and hamper his or her ability to resist intense impulses to take drugs. Fortunately, treatments are available to help people counter addiction's powerful disruptive effects. Research shows that combining addiction treatment medications with behavioral therapy is the best way to ensure success for most patients. Treatment approaches that are tailored to each patient's drug abuse patterns and any co-occurring medical, psychiatric, and social problems can lead to sustained recovery and a life without drug abuse. Similar to other chronic, relapsing diseases, such as diabetes, asthma or heart disease, drug addiction can be managed successfully: as with other chronic diseases, it is not uncommon for a person to relapse and begin abusing drugs again. Relapse, however, does not signal treatment failure-rather, it indicates that treatment should be reinstated or adjusted or that an alternative treatment is needed to help the individual regain control and recover.

Drugs contain chemicals that tap into the brain's communication system and disrupt the way nerve cells normally send, receive, and process information. There are at least two ways that drugs cause this disruption, by imitating the brain's natural chemical messengers and by over-stimulating the "reward circuit" of the brain. Some drugs (marijuana and heroin) have a similar structure to chemical messengers called neurotransmitters, which are naturally produced by the brain. This similarity allows the drugs to "fool" the brain's receptors and activate nerve cells to send abnormal messages. Other drugs, such as cocaine or methamphetamine, can cause the nerve cells to release abnormally large amounts of natural neurotransmitters (mainly dopamine) or to prevent the normal recycling of these brain chemicals, which is needed to shut off the signaling between neurons. The result is a brain awash in dopamine, a neurotransmitter present in brain regions that control movement, emotion, motivation and feelings of pleasure. The overstimulation of this reward system, which normally responds to natural behaviors linked to survival (eating, spending time with loved ones, etc.), produces euphoric effects in response to psychoactive drugs. This reaction sets in motion a reinforcing pattern that "teaches" people to repeat the rewarding behavior of abusing drugs.

As a person continues to abuse drugs, the brain adapts to the overwhelming surges in dopamine by producing less dopamine or by reducing the number of dopamine receptors in the reward circuit. The result is a lessening of dopamine's impact on the reward circuit, which reduces the abuser's ability to enjoy not only the drugs but also other events in life that previously brought pleasure. This decrease compels the addicted person to keep abusing drugs in an attempt to bring the dopamine function back to normal, but now larger amounts of the drug are required to achieve the same dopamine high- an effect known as tolerance. Long – term abuse causes changes in other brain chemical systems and circuits as well Glutamate is a neurotransmitter that influences the reward circuit and the ability to learn. When the optimal concentration of glutamate is altered by drug abuse, the brain attempts to compensate, which can impair cognitive function. Brain imaging studies of drug – addicted individuals show changes in areas of the brain that are critical to judgment, decision making, learning, memory and behaviour control. Together, these changes can drive an abuser to seek out and take drugs compulsively despite adverse, even devastating consequences- that is the nature of addiction.

No single factor can predict whether a person will become addicted to drugs. Risk for addiction is influenced by a combination of factors that include individual biology, social environment, and age or stage of development. The more rick factors an individual has, the greater the chance that taking drugs can lead to addiction.

Biology: The genes that people are born with- in combination with environmental influences- account for about half of their addiction vulnerability. Additionally, gender, ethnicity, and the presence of other mental disorders may influence risk for drug abuse and addiction.

Environment: A person's environment includes many different influences, from family and friends to socioeconomic status and quality of life in general. Factors such as peer pressure, physical and sexual abuse, stress, and quality of parenting can greatly influence the occurrence of drug abuse and the escalation to addiction in a person's life.

Development: Genetic and environmental factors interact with critical development stages in a person's life to affect addiction vulnerability. Although taking drugs at any age can lead to addiction, the earlier that drug use begins, the more likely it will progress to more serious abuse, which poses a special challenge to adolescents. Because areas in their brains that govern decision making, judgment, and self-control are still developing, adolescents may be especially prone to risk-taking behaviours.

Prevention is the key: Drug addiction is a preventable disease, results from research have shown that prevention programs involving families, schools, communities, and the media are effective in reducing drug abuse. Although many events and cultural factors affect drug abuse trends, when youths perceive drug abuse as harmful, drug addiction can be prevented. Talk to your children about their concerns. Help with the little things; that way you will always be one step ahead of the game.

Aspartame is the most controversial food additive in history, and its approval for use in food was the most contested in FDA history. The artificial sweetener was approved, not on scientific grounds, but rather because of strong political and financial pressure, after all, aspartame was previously listed by the pentagon as a biochemical warfare agent! It is hard to believe such a chemical would be allowed into the food supply, but it was, and has been wreaking silent havoc with people's health for the past 35 years. The truth is it should never have been released onto the market, and allowing it to remain in the food chain is seriously hurting people- no matter how many times you rebrand it under a fancy new name.

The deceptive marketing of aspartame: it is sold commercially under names line NutraSweet, Canderel, and now Amino Sweet, aspartame can be found in more than 6,000 foods, including soft drinks, chewing gum, table-top sweeteners, diet and diabetic foods, breakfast cereals, jams, sweets, vitamins, prescriptions and over the counter drugs. Aspartame producer Ajinomoto chose to rebrand it under the name Amino sweet, to "remind the industry that aspartame tastes just like sugar, and that it's made from amino acids- the building blocks of protein that are abundant in our diet". This is deception at its finest: begin with a shred of truth, and then spin it to fit your own agenda. In this case, the agenda is to make you believe that aspartame is somehow a harmless, natural sweetener made with two amino acids that are essential for health and present in your diet already. They want you to believe aspartame delivers all the benefits of sugar and none of its drawbacks. But nothing could be further from the truth.

How aspartame wreaks havoc on your health

Did you know there have been more reports to the FDA for aspartame reactions than for all other food additives combined? While a variety of symptoms have been reported, almost two- thirds of them fall into the neurological and behavioral category consisting mostly of headaches, mood alterations and hallucinations. The remaining third is mostly gastrointestinal symptoms. This chart will familiarize you with some of the terrifying side-effects and health problems you could encounter if you consume products containing this chemical. Unfortunately, aspartame toxicity is not well-known by doctors, despite its frequency. Diagnosis is also hampered by the fact that it mimics several other common health conditions, such as: Multiple sclerosis, Parkinson's disease, Alzheimer's disease, Fibromyalgia, Arthritis, Multiple chemical sensitivity, Chronic fatigue syndrome, Attention deficit disorder, Panic disorder, Depression and other psychological disorders, lupus, Diabetes and diabetic complications, Birth defects, Lymphoma, Lyme disease, Hypothyroidism.

In recent years, food manufactures have increasingly focused on developing low-calorie foods and drinks to help you maintain a healthy weight and avoid obesity. Unfortunately, the science behind these products is so flawed; most of these products can actually lead to increased weight gain. Research has discovered that drinking diet soda increases your risk of metabolic syndrome, and may double your risk of obesity; the complete opposite of the stated intention behind these "zero calories" drinks. The sad truth is that diet food and drinks ruin your body's ability to count calories, stimulate your appetite, thus boosting your inclination to overindulge.

Most public health agencies and a lot of nutritionists, recommend these toxic artificial sweeteners as an acceptable alternative to sugar, which is at best confusing and at worst harming the health of those who take their misguided advice. Truly, there is enough evidence showing the dangers of consuming artificial sweeteners to fill an entire book-. If you or your loved ones drink diet beverages or eat diet foods, this will explain how you have been deceived about the truth behind artificial sweeteners like aspartame and sucralose- for greed, profits and at the expense of your health. Almost two-thirds of all documented side effects of aspartame consumption are neurological. One of the reasons for this side effect, researchers have discovered, is because the phenylalanine in aspartame dissociates from the ester bond. While these amino acids are indeed completely natural and safe, they were never designed to be ingested as isolated amino acids in massive quantities, which will cause complications. This will also increase dopamine levels in your brain; this can lead to symptoms of depression because it distorts your serotonin\dopamine balance. It can also lead to migraine headaches and brain tumors through a similar mechanism.

The aspartic acid in aspartame is a well-documented excitotoxin. Excitotoxins are usually amino acids, such as glutamate and aspartate. These special amino acids cause particular brain cells to become excessively excited, to the point they die. Excitotoxins can also cause a loss of brain synapses and connecting fiber. A review conducted in 2008 found that consuming a lot of aspartame may inhibit the ability of enzymes in your brain to function normally, and may lead to neurodegeneration. According to researchers, consuming a lot of aspartame can disturb: the metabolism of amino acids, protein structure and metabolism, the integrity of nucleic acids, neuronal function, endocrine balances. Furthermore, the ester bond in aspartame breaks down to formaldehyde and methanol, which are also toxic. So it is not surprising that this popular artificial sweetener has also been found to cause cancer.

If you suffer from sweet cravings, it's easy to convince yourself you're doing the right thing by opting for a zero calorie sweetener like aspartame. Please understand that you will do more harm than good to your body this way. It is important to realize that your body craves sweets when you are not giving it the proper fuel it needs. If you are following a program at the beginning of the book you should be starting to feel full and satisfied. When you are fueling your body with good nutrition; you stop the sweet cravings significantly, and they may even disappear.

ZIKA VIRUS

Now this is a new one for us all: I have only started researching. This is what I have found out so far- these facts are from World Health Organization.

Zika virus disease is caused by a virus transmitted primarily by Aedes mosquitoes. People with Zika virus can have symptoms that can include mild fever, skin rash, conjunctivitis, muscle and joint pain, malaise or headache. These symptoms normally last for 2 to 7 days. There is no specific treatment or vaccine currently available. The best form of prevention is protection against mosquito bites. The virus is known to circulate in Africa, the Americas, Asia and the pacific.

Zika virus is an emerging mosquito-borne virus that was first identified in Uganda in 1947 in rhesus monkeys through a monitoring network of sylvatic yellow fever. It was subsequently identified in humans in 1952 in Uganda and the United Republic of Tanzania. Outbreaks of Zika virus have been recorded in Africa, the Americas, Asia and the pacific.

Signs and symptoms = the time from exposure to symptoms of Zika virus is not clear, but is likely to be a few days. The symptoms are similar to other arbovirus infections such as dengue, and include fever, skin rashes, conjunctivitis, muscle and joint pain, malaise, and headache.

Complications of Zika virus disease= during large outbreaks in French Polynesia and Brazil in 2013 and 2015; national health authorities reported potential neurological and auto-immune complications of Zika virus disease. Recently in Brazil local health authorities have observed an increase in Guillain-Barre syndrome which coincided with Zika virus infections in the general public, as well as an increase in babies born with microcephaly in north east Brazil. Substantial new research has strengthened the association between Zika infection and the occurrence of fetal malformations and neurological disorders; however, more investigation is needed to better understand the relationship. Other potential causes are also being investigated. Like maybe GMOs! Transmission = Zika virus is transmitted to people through the bite of an infected mosquito from the Aedes genus, mainly Aedes aegypti in tropical regions. This is the same mosquito that transmits dengue, chikungunya and yellow fever. However sexual transmission of Zika virus is also possible. Other modes of transmission such as blood transfusion and perinatal transmission are currently being investigated. Zika virus disease outbreaks were reported for the first time from the pacific in 2007 and 2013 (Yap and French Polynesia, respectively), and in 2015 from the Americas (Brazil and Colombia) and Africa (Cabo Verde). In total 64 countries and territories have reported transmission of Zika virus since 1st January 2007.

Diagnosis = infection with Zika virus may be suspected based on symptoms and recent history of travel (residence or travel to an area where Zika virus is known to be present). Zika virus diagnosis can only be confirmed by laboratory testing for the presence of Zika virus RNA in the blood or other body fluids, such as urine or saliva.

Prevention = mosquitoes and their breeding sites pose a significant risk factor for Zika virus infection. Prevention and control relies on reducing mosquitoes through source reduction (removal and modification of breeding sites) and reducing contact between mosquitoes and people. This can be done by using insect repellent regularly; wearing clothes(preferably light-coloured) that cover as much of the body as possible; installing physical barriers such as window screens in buildings, closed doors and windows, and if needed, additional personal protection, such as sleeping under mosquito nets during the day. It is extremely important to empty, clean or cover containers regularly that can store water, such as buckets, drums, pots, etc. other mosquito breeding sites should be cleaned or removed including flowerpots, used tyres and roof gutters. Communities must support the efforts of the local government to reduce the density of mosquitoes in their locality. Efforts must be made to eliminate mosquito breeding sites such as still water soon after rains and its accumulation in discarded containers and waste materials in and around houses.

Repellents should contain DEET and product label should be strictly followed. During outbreaks, health authorities may advise that spraying of insecticides be carried out. Insecticides recommended by the pesticide evaluation scheme may also be used as larvicides to treat relatively large water containers. Travellers should take the basic precautions to protect themselves from mosquito bites.

Sexual transmission of Zika virus is possible. All people who have been infected with Zika virus and their sexual partners should practice safer sex, by using condoms correctly and consistently. Pregnant women's sex partners living in or returning from areas where local transmission of Zika virus occurs should practice safer sex. In addition, people returning from areas where local transmission of Zika virus occurs should adopt safer sexual practices or consider abstinence for at least four weeks after their return to reduce the risk of onward transmission.

Treatment= Zika virus disease is usually relatively mild and requires no specific treatment. People sick with Zika virus should get plenty of rest, drink lots of fluids, and treat pain and fever with common medicines. If symptoms worsen, you should seek medical care and advice. There is no vaccine currently available.

Zika has been linked to dangerous neurological birth disorder in newborns. The Zika virus, transmitted by the aggressive Aedes aegypti mosquito, has spread to at least 34 countries and territories: WHO estimates 3 to 4 million people across the Americas will be infected with the virus in the next year. The U.S. Centers for disease control and prevention is warning pregnant women against traveling to those areas: health officials in several of those countries are telling women to avoid pregnancy and in some cases for up to two years. Zika is commanding attention because of an alarming connection between the virus and microcephaly, a neurological disorder that results in babies being born with abnormally small heads. It causes severe developmental issues and sometimes death. Since October, Brazil has seen 508 confirmed cases of microcephaly in newborns. At least seventeen of those cases have a confirmed link to the Zika virus. There were only 146 cases in 2014; so far 27 babies have died from the condition, with at least five linked to Zika. An additional 70 deaths are under investigation, and authorities are investigating 3,935 suspected cases.

Other Latin Countries are seeing cases in newborns as well. Colombia reported more than 6,000 pregnant women have tested positive for the virus, while in the United States one Hawaiian baby was born with microcephaly linked to the Zika virus after his mother returned from

Brazil. Health officials are looking at a couple of first trimester miscarriages among women who had traveled to infected areas and became ill. They can't say with certainty whether Zika caused the pregnancy losses. More than 20 states have confirmed the virus in individuals who traveled to areas where the virus is circulating. Some states are following pregnant women with the virus. In most people, symptoms of the virus are mild, including fever, headache, rash and possible pink eye. In fact 80% of those infected never know they have the disease. That's especially concerning for pregnant women, as this virus has now been shown to pass through amniotic fluid to the growing baby. We now know that fetuses can be infected with the virus. That's not new for infectious diseases, but it is new for this virus.

The virus is most commonly transmitted when an Aedes mosquito bites a person with an active infection and then spreads the virus by biting others. Those people become carriers when they have symptoms. In February the CDC reported the first case of locally acquired Zika virus in the United States in this outbreak, it was not from a mosquito bite. Instead it was passed via sex. The individual has sex with a partner who had recently returned from Venezuela infected with the mosquito-borne virus. The patient had not traveled. Federal and state health officials are investigating more than a dozen cases of possible sexual transmission of the virus, some of them among pregnant women. This could mean sexual transmission is more likely than previously thought according to the CDC. The virus is in the blood for about a week. How long it would remain in the semen is something that needs to be studied. Previously, there had been only three documented cases linking Zika to sex. During a 2013 outbreak in French Polynesia, semen and urine samples from a 44 year old Tahitian man tested positive for Zika even when blood samples did not. A second documented case in the United Kingdom in 2014 found high levels of the Zika virus in semen up to 62 days after the onset of the illness; in fact the viral load was stronger at that time than when the first samples were taken. Even earlier, in 2008 Brian Foy a microbiologist contracted Zika after travel to Senegal; his wife came down with the disease a few days later even though she had not left northern Colorado and was not exposed to any mosquitoes carrying the virus. The CDC noted: "there have been no reports of sexual transmission of Zika virus from infected women to their sex partners." The CDC said there have been documented cases of virus transmission during labor, blood transfusion and laboratory exposure. While Zika has been found in breast milk, it is not yet confirmed it can be passed to a baby through nursing.

The FDA has taken measures to protect the U. S. blood supply by asking individuals who have returned from infected areas to defer donating blood for four weeks after their return. If they have had symptoms of the virus, they are asked to hold off and if they have had sexual contact with someone who has returned from travel. Canadian Blood Services and the Red Cross have made similar recommendations. The CDC said while research continues on sex and other avenues of transmission, the "vast majority of spread" of the Zika virus is going to be from mosquitoes.

Where is the Zika virus now? The Zika virus is now being transmitted is Aruba, Barbados, Bolivia, Bonaire, Brazil, Colombia, Puerto Rico, Costa Rica, Curacao, Dominican Republic, Ecuador, El Salvador, French Guiana, Guadeloupe, Guatemala, Guyana, Haiti, Honduras, Jamaica, Marshall Islands, Martinique, Mexico, Nicaragua, Panama, Paraguay, Saint Martin, Suriname, Trinidad and Tobago, U.S. Virgin Islands, Venezuela, American Samoa, Samoa, Tonga and Cape Verde, according to the CDC and WHO.

Zika has arrived in the United States from travelers returning from these infected areas and, in one confirmed case and 14 suspected cases, through sexual transmission. The concern, of course, is whether imported cases could result in more locally transmitted cases within your country.

The Asian tiger mosquito, which along with Aedes aegypti transmits Zika virus, is present in many parts off the United States. If mosquitoes in the United States do become carriers, a model created by Toronto researchers found more than 63% of the U.S. population lives in areas where Zika virus might spread during seasonally warm months. A little more than 7% of Americans live in areas where the cold might not kill of the mosquito in the winter, leaving them vulnerable year- round.

With no treatment or vaccine available, the only protection against Zika is to avoid travel to areas with an active infestation. If you do travel to a country where Zika is present, the CDC advises strict adherence to mosquito protection measures: Use an EPA – approved repellent over sunscreen, were long pants and long-sleeve shirts thick enough to block a mosquito bite, and sleep in air-conditioned, screened rooms.

If you have Zika, you can keep from spreading it to others by avoiding mosquito bites during the first week of illness. The female Aedes aegypti, the primary carrier of Zika, is an aggressive biter, preferring daytime to dusk and indoors to outdoors. Keeping screens on windows and doors is critical to preventing entry to homes and hotel rooms. For women of childbearing age, the CDC now recommends discussing, "strategies to prevent unintended (pregnancies) Including counseling on family planning and the correct and consistent use of effective contraceptive methods in the context of the potential risks of Zika virus transmission". The CDC also called on local health officials to implement routine testing recommendations for pregnant women with or without symptoms based on local transmission of the virus and their capacity to process them. Researchers around the world are working very hard trying to create a Zika vaccine. A clinical trial for a Zika virus vaccine could begin this year. WHO says it will be at least 18 months until large-scale clinical trials get underway.

While in development, it is important to understand we will not have a vaccine this year or even in the next few years. Studies show local control is only marginally effective since it is hard to get to all possible breeding areas. Since Aedes aegypti has evolved to live near humans and "can replicate in flower vases and other tiny sources of water," the mosquitoes are difficult to find and eradicate.

Zika virus in now in Canada

On march 24th 2016: the case of a woman who was believed to have contracted the virus; after having sex with a man who had travelled to a country where Zika is prevalent. To date there have been 55 other confirmed cases of Zika among Canadians, all of whom were infected while travelling to regions where the disease is spreading, including South and Central America, parts of Mexico and the Caribbean. Among them are two B.C. women, who are pregnant. While bites from infected mosquitoes remain the primary way to get Zika virus, sexual transmission of the virus is to be expected given that a small number of cases have been reported elsewhere in the world. Most people who contract the infection have no symptoms; those who do get sick experience such ill effects as fever, joint pain, rash and red eyes. The disease usually resolves in about a week. However, the virus had been potentially linked in Brazil to thousands of cases of abnormally small heads in infants born to women who were infected while pregnant. After months of intensive research, scientists confirmed earlier this month that Zika does cause what is known as microcephaly as well as other fetal brain defects. There also has been a spike in cases of Guillain-Barre syndrome, a neurological condition that can cause muscle weakness or even partial paralysis, among Zika-infected children and adults.

Zika was first detected in a rhesus monkey in the Zika forest of Uganda in 1947. Since then the disease has spread from Africa and Southeast Asia, across the Pacific to South America and beyond.

PHAC said there have been no confirmed cases of locally acquired Zika from infected mosquitoes, as the species that transmit the virus are not established in Canada, making the risk to Canadians "very low".

However, the agency said pregnant women and those planning a pregnancy should avoid travel to countries with Zika outbreaks. If travel cannot be avoided or postponed, strict mosquito- bite prevention measures should be taken because of the risk of serious health effects on the unborn baby.

Travellers returning from Zika – affected countries and their sexual partners need to take precautions to protect against transmission:

Women planning a pregnancy are strongly advised to wait at least two months before trying to conceive to ensure any possible Zika infection has cleared from the body.

Because the Zika virus can persist in semen for an extended period, infected men are advised to use condoms with a pregnant partner for the duration of the pregnancy. Infected men should use condoms with any partner for six months to prevent sexual transmission of the virus.

PANDAS: A SCARY AND CONTROVERSIAL DISORDER

Could a sudden, severe change in a child's behavior be brought on by something as common as strep throat? Many experts and distraught parents say yes. So what is going on, and which children are at risk.

Pandas: first identified in 1998 by investigators at the National Institute of Mental Health, including pediatrician Susan Swedo M.D., now chief of the pediatrics and developmental neuroscience branch. In the 1980s, Dr. Swedo was among those studying a neurological disease called Sydenham's chorea, marked by involuntary jerky movements; that occur in up to 20 to 30 percent of children who have acute rheumatic fever, a rare illness caused by a strep infection. When the NIMH investigators began studying children who had severe, sudden- onset OCD, without the jerking movements, they discovered that many of the children had recently had a strep infection. If strep was known to cause one neurological illness, researchers reasoned, it might cause another.

How does Pandas take hold? A bacterial infection such as strep triggers the immune system to produce antibodies; but instead of attacking the infection, they go after the basal ganglia, the part of the brain that controls emotions, behaviors, and physical movements, and the result is OCD –like behaviors and /or tics. One distinguishing feature of PANDAS is the abrupt onset of symptoms. Typically, OCD develops over years or months, but in Pandas the symptoms literally begin overnight. While there's no test to detect Pandas, research published in the journal of Pediatrics found that, compared to children who have typical OCD, those diagnosed with Pandas were more likely to have biological evidence of a recent strep infection, a sudden onset of psychiatric symptoms, and an easing of those symptoms while taking antibiotics.

Pandas: also have its skeptics, who see it as more of a hypothesis than a real disorder. One is neurologist director of the movement disorders program at Atlantic Neuroscience Institute at Overlook Medical Center, in Summit, New Jersey. He calls studies linking strep and Pandas flawed, contending that their evidence has been mostly anecdotal and unreliable. "It's not uncommon for tics and OCD to wax and wane," he says. Parents often take their child to the doctor when his or her symptoms have peaked, he adds, so the fact that they subside after treatment with antibiotics does not prove anything. He isn't convinced that symptoms come on as suddenly as parents report, either. Most children diagnosed with Pandas, he says, have had prior tics or obsessive-compulsive symptoms, often for months or years. "The so called onset is just more severe." This begs the question. Why is Pandas linked to strep? "Because strep is extremely common, it can be connected to almost anything.

This is for moms and dads who have dedicated their lives to raising awareness about this disorder- you are the silent heroes to countless children.

For every parent of a child with an illness, especially a mental illness, there is a particular story. But when you meet a parent of a child with PANDAS (typically a child between ages 3 – 14 you will hear the same panicked story over and over. A child who was happy at home and at school, and was social and athletic, is now walking in circles for hours, washing hands until they bleed, asking the same questions over and over. A child that used to be comforted by a hug is now inconsolable. They may be begging parents for help, begging for a way to end the horror that exists only in their minds. Imagine a child screaming in terror in a corner, and a parent unable to hold them. These parents will tell you in detail about the day or week that their child changed. Children may exhibit some or all of these symptoms.

Acute sudden onset of OCD, challenges with eating, and at the extreme end anorexia, sensory issues such as sensitivity to clothes, sound, and light, handwriting noticeably deteriorates, urinary frequency or bedwetting, small motor skills deteriorate- a craft project from yesterday is now impossible to complete, tics, inattentive, distractible, unable to focus and has difficulties with memory, overnight onset of anxiety or panic attacks over things that were no big deal a few days ago, such as thunderstorms or bugs, suddenly unable to separate from their caregiver, or to sleep alone, screaming for hours on end, fear of germs and other more traditional-looking OCD symptoms. You will often find these parents on the computer every night, desperate for an explanation that makes sense. They are seeking specialists who can help- and finding no answers. They are starting to feel crazy themselves, because no one seems to believe what they are going through.

How to identify pandas in your child; sudden dramatic onset is the most salient characteristic and differentiates pandas from a more frequent pediatric OCD presentation- which involves subclinical symptoms becoming gradually more severe. Incapacitating fears and anxieties seem to come on "overnight" with many parents being able to name the exact day when their child changed. In addition, while the mean age of OCD in children is between 9 and 10, Pandas can start at a younger age such as 5 or 6, often corresponding with a diagnosis of strep. Doctors are encouraged to assess for: A history of sore throat, fever, exudative pharyngitis, cervical adenopathy (enlarged and tender lymph nodes in the neck), enlarged or damaged tonsils, a typical presentation of strep, especially in young children, include abdominal pain and vomiting, vaginal or perianal redness. In some cases of Pandas, the strep appeared to be "hiding" in the sinuses or middle ear resulting in a negative throat culture. It is also possible that non-strep organisms can cause a similar neuropsychiatric illness in vulnerable children. Therefore, it is important to check for mycoplasma, mono, or exposure to Lyme disease. During a meeting in 2010, researchers and clinicians across the country discussed current Pandas criteria defining this devastating illness in children. And additional category, pediatric acute-onset neuropsychiatric syndrome (PANS), was defined. This definition allows researchers to study pediatric patients often seen in doctor's offices; a child who comes down with severe sudden onset OCD as the primary symptom, sometimes triggered by infections other than strep. Research into this focused group of children may then be translated into treatment for many kinds of sudden onset infectious triggered mental illness Pandas still exists as a research definition.

Medical professionals should look for: Abrupt, dramatic onset of OCD is the first diagnostic criterion for PANS. Children may have mild "quirks" or even some signs of OCD prior to this abrupt dramatic onset. Mild micro-episodes may have occurred in the past. However, in the space of a few days, they "fall of a cliff" dramatically; causing a significant decrease in the child's ability to function. Impairment is significant. Parents can usually name the day that the crisis occurred and have vivid memories of the first obsessions or compulsions because of their extreme nature. As an example, a normally joyful, balanced emotionally, independent, social child may turn into a child that has extreme temper tantrums that are out of character, and can no longer leave a parent's side without accommodation. Panic attacks and unusual anxieties are not uncommon. In addition to the typical obsessional fears and compulsive behaviors, this criterion also may be satisfied by the sudden severe onset of food avoidance, anorexia and eating restrictions. These occur as solitary symptoms among PANS patients, as well as from complications resulting from obsessional fears of choking, vomiting or of contaminated foods. Although there appears to be uniformity in the acuity and severity of onset of the co-occurring symptoms, there is great variability in the nature of the symptoms accompanying the OCD. As a result, the second major criterion for PANS is the concurrent acute onset of additional symptoms from at least two of the following seven categories: 1. Anxiety (particularly acute separation anxiety and irrational fears). 2. Emotional liability and / or depression. 3. Irritability, aggression and/or oppositional behaviors. 4. Behavioral (developmental) regression. 5. Sudden deterioration in school performance. 6. Sensory or motor abnormalities (particularly dysgraphia/ trouble with handwriting). 7. Somatic/ physical signs and symptoms. As in most of psychiatry, PANS is a clinical diagnosis, meaning that there are currently no laboratory or genetic tests that can confirm the diagnosis. As such, a second opinion to find consensus on the diagnosis of PANS between tow experienced physicians may be useful.

Many physicians report that a throat culture appears to be key (even if there are no signs or symptoms of pharyngitis) due to the difficulty in properly sampling these children, a two – swab sample should be taken to check for bacterial colonization. The first swab should be a rapid strep test. It is very important that the culture is obtained properly by vigorously swabbing across the entire pharynx, behind both tonsils and the uvula. If the child doesn't gag and protest, the swab is probably inadequate. If negative, use the second swab for a 4- hour agar plate culture. If these are both negative, consider testing for Lyme disease, Mycoplasma, vitamin D, Ferritin and thyroid. Many children with recurrent upper respiratory infections have immune deficiencies and would benefit from an immune function assessment such as blood counts measuring quantitative immunoglobulins and a referral to a pediatric immunologist. Many physicians rely on antibodies to the exotoxins of streptococcus to confirm a prior infection measuring ASO and AntiDNaseB. These tests have fixed windows where the measurement may begin to be positive 1-8 weeks after initial infection. Typically two measurements are required. The first should be obtained as soon as possible after the suspected infection and the second at least six weeks later. It is currently unknown whether carrying the bacteria without an active infection alone is sufficient to cause symptoms in PANS children.

While acknowledging the need for additional research, we also cannot sit by while children scream in terror. We have to help children suffering today. Best practices suggest that you develop a treatment plan based on interventions with the minimum effective dose, and intervention with the best cost/benefit ratio (less intrusive, minimal short term and long term side effects, good at preventing relapse, easy to administer and tolerated well). Treatments that have the best research behind them; at this point in time PANDAS and PANS treatments are drastically under researched.

The original research studies investigating possible treatment options were done by giving children IVIG (intravenous immunoglobin) this treatment gives the child antibodies from a myriad of donors. Researchers don't exactly know how IVIC works, but it appears to help in a number of autoimmune illnesses.

In PANDAS, IVIG reduced the OCD symptoms severity for 82% of children suspected of having Pandas. While IVIG is considered quite safe for treating auto-immune disorders, there are several risks, which I would like to make you aware off. (Nausea, vomiting, and headache are not uncommon and in rare instances, aseptic meningitis, or allergic reactions may occur). Although most side effects are not harmful in the long term, they are unpleasant and therefore IVIG therapy is generally recommended only for severe or persistent cases for immune deficiency disorders. Research shows that using antibiotics as a prophylaxis to prevent strep successfully reduces neuropsychiatric exacerbations. Another study will soon start collaboration between Harvard and the University of South Florida; they will be examining a common treatment course successfully used by clinicians: using antibiotics in children with PANDAS. Early in the disease if strep is present, this is an obvious course. But no research has yet been done on why many clinicians find that a longer term course of antibiotics often seems to offer great hope to families suffering from this disease; even after the actual triggering illness is over. Some physicians have found the following particularly helpful for new, sudden onset cases.

Use antibiotics for 3-6 weeks initially. Use of Augmentin has anecdotally been found to be more effective at a relatively high dose as well as the Cephalosporin's (cephalexin, cefdinir) and azithromycin. Consider using probiotics but not at the same time of day; allow 2-3 hours in between. If no improvement is seen after 3-4 weeks, a physician may consider an alternate class of antibiotic treatment. If symptoms completely remit, a trial off the antibiotic may be attempted. If symptoms return, additional treatment may be warranted. In many cases, a physician will see a child several weeks after the initial onset, or in a second exacerbation. In that case, some clinicians have recommended the following: a throat culture can still be very informative at this point as well as antibody levels. Then treat with antibiotics while waiting for the results. If there is a marked reduction in symptoms, gradually wean. With a recurrence, antibiotics are reintroduced and continued as needed. Try to gather retrospective information, ask for detailed pediatrician records to be forwarded and nail down the exact timing of testing and labs since prior testing may have been limited, a trial of antibiotic appears to be low risk.

Cognitive behavior therapy or (CBT) unlike traditional onset OCD, where research clearly guides a mental health and medical professional's decision about how to proceed with treatment, PANS onset OCD is still under researched. As we wait for studies to be completed we still need to develop treatment strategies that can address the pain and suffering of children and families now. For many PANS children the suddenness of onset ant the migratory nature of the obsessions/compulsions can make exposure and response prevention therapy challenging: a combination of a medical intervention and traditional ERP might be the might be the best course of action at this point. For some children an initial treatment with antibiotics or IVIG results in significant relief of symptoms. For those with slow or partial remission of symptoms, ensuring that EPR is included seems to be critical. Children develop habits and fears quickly and they may use EPR treatment to teach their brain to ignore the irrational fear signals they have been receiving. EPR teaches a child concrete tools to overcome OCD thoughts on a daily basis. Many doctors find that learning EPR allows the entire family to function more calmly during future exacerbations, while seeking medical help. Some recent but preliminary work found strong effects for this approach in children with PANDAS.

Most doctors experienced in treating children with PANDAS do not initially recommend SSRIs, especially given the very young age of many of the children.

In the absence of research, something has to be done to help these children, their suffering is intense. And the risk of long-term damage cannot be ignored. One prospective study conducted in a pediatrician's office suggests that first- onset PANDAS symptoms may remit following successful treatment of the strep infection with antibiotics. There where know follow-up reports on these children, so it is unknown if some experienced a second exacerbation following successful treatment of the initial onset of PANDAS symptoms.

Printed in the United States
By Bookmasters